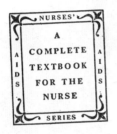

NURSES'

A
COMPLETE
TEXTBOOK
FOR THE
NURSE

AIDS

AIDS

SERIES

AIDS TO HYGIENE
FOR NURSES

AIDS TO HYGIENE
FOR NURSES

A Textbook of Personal and Communal Health

by

EDITH M. FUNNELL
S.R.N., D.N. (London)
*Formerly Sister Tutor, Royal Sussex County
Hospital, Brighton*

with a Foreword by
CLEMENT MUIR
M.B., Ch.B., M.R.C.P., D.P.H.
*Deputy Senior Administrative Medical Officer
North-West Metropolitan Regional Hospital Board*

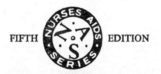

FIFTH EDITION

LONDON
BAILLIÈRE, TINDALL AND COX
7 AND 8 HENRIETTA STREET, W.C.2
Reprinted 1958

First Edition, June 1938
Second Edition, June 1940
Reprinted, November 1940
Reprinted, June 1941
Reprinted, February 1942
Reprinted, July 1942
Reprinted, January 1943
Reprinted, February 1944
Reprinted, September 1944
Reprinted, November 1945
Reprinted, October 1946
Reprinted, July 1947
Third Edition, November 1948
Fourth Edition, June 1950
Reprinted, June 1951
Reprinted, February 1953
Reprinted, June 1954
Reprinted, January 1955
Reprinted, March 1955
Reprinted, September 1955
Fifth Edition, September 1956
Reprinted, April 1958

Printed in Great Britain

FOREWORD

TO

THE NURSES' AIDS SERIES

The Nurses' Aids Series is designed to provide a series of textbooks in the various fields of knowledge required by the modern nurse. It covers the subjects included in the syllabus of the General parts of the Register, and, in addition, includes volumes on certain specialized subjects such as fevers, tropical nursing, the setting of trays and trolleys, and theatre technique. New volumes are added to the Series from time to time.

Each volume is a complete textbook on its subject (the title "Aids to" indicates that the books are aids to knowledge and not aids to the study of larger books) and is written, except in a few instances, by a Sister Tutor at a prominent hospital. The whole Series aims at providing concisely, clearly and simply just that quantity of information which the nurse needs to possess, gathered together in well-illustrated, easily read and easily carried volumes at a price within the means of any nurse. Judged by the welcome the whole Series has received, this aim has been accomplished, and the student nurse has at her disposal a set of convenient, up-to-date, comprehensive textbooks.

The General Editors would like to take this opportunity of thanking all those who have been so helpful in their criticism and support of the Series.

(*Signed*) KATHARINE F. ARMSTRONG, S.R.N., S.C.M., D.N.(London) (*formerly Sister Tutor at King's College Hospital, London, and Editor of the "Nursing Times"*).

MARJORIE HOUGHTON, M.B.E., S.R.N., S.C.M., D.N. (London) (*Education Officer, General Nursing Council; formerly Sister Tutor at University College Hospital, London*).

E. JOAN BOCOCK, S.R.N., S.C.M., D.N. (London) (*Principal Tutor at the Royal Free Hospital, London; formerly Sister Tutor at St. Thomas's Hospital, London*).

WINIFRED L. HUNTLY, S.R.N., S.C.M., D.N.(London) (*Principal Tutor at the Royal Masonic Hospital*).

NORMA JAMIESON, M.A., S.R.N., S.C.M., (*Sister Tutor at St. Thomas's Hospital, London*).

LONDON   GENERAL EDITORS

FOREWORD TO FIFTH EDITION

Hygiene is something we accept as part of our daily life
and without as a rule enquiring into the whys and
wherefores. It is, however, fundamental to civilized life
for man to take such steps as are known to him to prevent disease and to promote health. The great com-
munities in cities and towns could not exist without the
constant vigilance of that body of people who concern
themselves with the safeguarding of health. Nor are
matters static; new discoveries are made yearly of factors deleterious to health, as for example, the dangers of
smoke pollution of the atmosphere, and the production
of "smog", and, once discovered, attempts are made to
prevent their ill effects. Even more recently the new
vaccine against poliomyelitis has been used in this
country with a view to preventing the occurrence of that
disease in the more susceptible ages.

This book provides an introduction to the subject of
preventive medicine and in my view admirably explains
this intricate subject. Miss Funnell, the authoress, has
a long and distinguished record as a teacher and she has
had remarkable success in this book in conveying her
knowledge in a clear and lucid manner. A fifth edition
within a few years indicates that in the past the book has
fulfilled a want. I am certain that this new edition will
prove quite as successful and impart to further genera-
tions of nurses the elementary facts about hygiene without which their training would be useless and their
education incomplete. While primarily written for
nurses, I have no hesitation in recommending it to a
much wider audience.

CLEMENT MUIR

LONDON
  May 1956

PREFACE TO FIFTH EDITION

It has been a very great pleasure to me that my small book on hygiene has proved so useful to student nurses. A further edition has now become necessary following the recent changes in the syllabus of the General Nursing Council as a result of which greater stress is laid on "Communal Health".

In order to give the student nurse a brief survey of the Public Health Services and the personnel which implements them it has been necessary to add much new material. To this end, in preparing this new edition, the order in which the subject matter is presented has been rearranged. The early chapters have been carefully revised and the later chapters (13 to 16) have been planned to deal exclusively with social aspects, covering Section XIII of the syllabus. It will be noted that the chapter on "Tropical Health" has been omitted, as this is dealt with in another volume in the Nurses' Aids series—*Aids to Tropical Nursing*.

A number of admirable illustrations from *Aids to Practical Hygiene* have been inserted in the text as it was felt that they would make it more interesting and attractive to the student nurse.

The plate section has been revised, new plates having replaced most of those in the previous edition. A wider selection has been made possible by the insertion in the text of the "Metropolitan Water Board" diagram in two colours.

To Miss Huntly I am very grateful for her advice and for reading the manuscript for me. To Dr. Clement Muir I offer my sincere thanks for his continued interest, advice and help, and to the publishers my gratitude for their kind assistance.

I hope the new edition will enable the book to continue as a suitable textbook for student nurses and will assist them in their training.   E. M. FUNNELL

BRIGHTON
May 1956

CONTENTS

Chapter   *Page*

INTRODUCTION xii

I. HOUSING AND HOME PLANNING . . 1

II. AIR AND VENTILATION 9

III. HEATING AND LIGHTING 30

IV. WATER SUPPLY 59

V. SANITATION: DRAINAGE AND REFUSE DISPOSAL 76

VI. HYGIENE OF THE INDIVIDUAL . . . 96

VII. HYGIENE OF THE FAMILY AT ALL AGES . 107

VIII. CLOTHING AND FABRICS 119

IX. INFECTION AND DISINFECTION: HYGIENE OF THE WARD AND SICK ROOM . . . 124

X. PARASITES AND HOUSE PESTS . . . 142

XI. FOOD AND FOOD VALUES . . . 169

XII. FOOD CONTAMINATION AND PRESERVATION . 201

XIII. SOCIAL SERVICES: ADMINISTRATION . 215

XIV. SOCIAL SERVICES: THE CHILDREN'S CHARTER 244

XV. SOCIAL SERVICES: SCHOOL AGE, OCCUPATIONAL HEALTH, OLD AGE . . . 251

XVI. PREVENTION AND CONTROL OF INFECTIOUS DISEASES 274

INDEX 295

INTRODUCTION

HYGIENE is the study of health, a very far-reaching subject, starting with the health of the individual, or Personal Hygiene, including in its wider aspect the health of the nation, or Public Health, and expanding ultimately to World Health.

The child as a rule is born healthy and with proper care and in a good environment remains so. There is very little inherited disease, although some individuals show less ability than others to thrive mentally and physically in unfavourable circumstances. The determining factor in most cases in deciding the course life will run is bound up in the environment in which the individual grows up, is educated, works, plays, mates and has children.

In considering living conditions we should include in our survey, the home, the climatic and sanitary conditions, food, educational arrangements, work places, recreational facilities and social relationships, including religious attachments. Hygiene, in the widest sense, is concerned with all of these.

CHAPTER I

HOUSING AND HOME PLANNING

Housing

In countries where populations are increasing the only way to keep abreast of the problem of housing is by meeting the yearly demand for new dwellings and at the same time maintaining existing premises in a state of good repair. When this aim is unattainable, as in times of war, the whole plan for efficient housing falls to pieces with resultant overcrowding, hardship and ill health (see p. 262). A report on satisfactory housing standards made after the second world war stresses the importance of a dry dwelling in good repair, well lighted and ventilated, with the following amenities: main water supply; provision for a hot water supply; a fixed bath and sink and facilities for laundering; a good drainage system with an internal water closet; heating facilities in each room and provision for fuel storage; sufficient points for artificial lighting; facilities for cooking and a ventilated larder.

In order to meet the demand for dwellings and to eliminate slums and overcrowding, new towns must be planned and built, extensions made to existing towns, and thousands of houses put into good repair, many of them being converted into flats.

The planning of a new town, or the extension of an existing town is a work of many aspects and great interest.

Having acquired the site, the first consideration is the *general lay out*, and the town planners whose aim it is to make a town of pleasing appearance, survey the site

1

and arrange to preserve, as far as they can, any beautiful natural features, such as trees and streams. The *road pattern* is made up of main and branch streets, squares and quadrangles. There are many ways of arranging these, but the main streets should always be wide and neither too curly nor too geometrical. They are often divided into dual traffic ways by concrete courses which, if made double with a foot or more of grass or flowers between them, add to the beauty of the street. Pavements should be really wide, with trees, kept carefully pruned, planted along the borders if possible. If the town design includes squares they can add much to the architectural effect. They often have grass centres, but paving is an alternative much used in some countries, with wooden or concrete tubs of flowers and shrubs, and wooden seats. This can be most attractive.

Open spaces in the town plan are large, and include parks and gardens, recreation and playing fields and children's playgrounds. In some towns these open spaces are arranged in an almost continuous pattern, to be within easy reach of all houses. As many trees as possible should be preserved and others planted.

Public buildings of all kinds should be centrally placed, as should also the shopping centre. Nursery schools need situating with special care with regard to traffic crossings. There should be plenty of space arranged for car parking in convenient sites.

With regard to *houses and dwellings*, the plan may include houses, detached, semi-detached or in terraces, and blocks of flats. Most people would prefer a detached house, with an individual garden, but in England, at least, this is not practicable in any large scale plan. Semi-detached and terrace houses generally have gardens, though perhaps small ones, but blocks of flats have communal gardens or none at all.

The *orientation of dwellings* is specially important, and sufficient space around is necessary for light and ventilation. Wide gaps should be arranged between high blocks of flats. *Lighting* includes both sunlight and daylight. Rooms facing between north-west and north-east are not suitable for living rooms or children's rooms, which should have a sunny aspect, whereas larders should always be on the shady side. Whatever the aspect of a room, it should be possible, for satisfactory daylight, to see the sky from most positions in it (except where trees grow close).

Gardens are one of the biggest arguments in favour of houses rather than flats. Divisions between them may be walls which are ideal but expensive, or perhaps fencing or hedges. In the front, very low walls or stone borders can give a charming effect, but any method is better than the iron railings of pre-war days. Paths to the house should be flagged or paved.

The House

The Walls. These should fulfil four functions. (1) They must be strong to carry the upper floors, and also durable; (2) They must be weather-proof and damp-proof, keeping out rain and snow and preventing ground damp from rising; (3) They should be insulated against the loss of heat from inside; (4) They should be insulated from noise.

Strong and durable modern houses are built with "cavity walls", that is two layers of bricks with a $2\frac{1}{4}$ inch cavity between, or hollow concrete blocks. The outside may be finished with a coat of plaster (a mixture of lime and cement), either smooth, roughcast, or pebbled, and this, together with the cavity, serves to make the house *weather-proof*. To prevent damp creeping up from below, a *damp-proof course* is inserted in the wall 6 inches above ground level and below the under side of any floor. It may be of sheet lead, slates in cement, asphalt, or a layer of bitumen on felt. A damp-proof course is also laid in parapets and chimney-stacks to prevent moisture from rain seeping downwards. Walls should be insulated from heat and noise.

Thermal Insulation. There are two ways of preventing loss of heat through walls and roofing or, alternatively, the penetration of heat from the atmosphere. One is the cavity in the walls which is a sealed air space and the other is the use of insulating boards. These are made of cork, fibre, asbestos, wood wool slabs or "blankets",

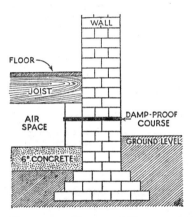

FIG. 1.—DIAGRAM OF WALL WITH DAMP-PROOF COURSE.

or roofing felt (see pp. 38–40). Whatever the method of heating the rooms, if it is carefully regulated, heat-insulation will save fuel expense.

Sound Insulation. This has become a problem of first importance due to ever increasing traffic noises, wireless and electrical equipment. Noise reduces efficiency in buildings where concentration is necessary, as in school class-rooms, and offices. It is also one of the chief objections to living in flats. Both outdoor and indoor noise must be considered. Outdoor noise is lessened by planning for lawns, trees, etc., between the building and the road; by arranging that rooms for work and study shall not face a noisy street; by the use of cavity walls, and above all by considerations of the windows. If the windows are open even a little way the room is hardly quieter than outside. A double window with screened ventilation openings is very satisfactory, and if it is plate glass it gives the best insulation possible. The drawback is that ventilation is not efficient, and the best solution is probably the fitting of extraction and intake fans. Indoor noise is difficult to eliminate. Plaster linings to walls are helpful, and for floor coverings carpets on underfelt or rubber carpets.

The Roof. If sloping (pitched), this is covered with slates, asbestos, cement slabs or tiles of various kinds. Corrugated iron has certain uses. Flat roofs are covered with copper, lead, zinc, bituminous felt or asphalt. Roofs are insulated by the same materials as walls.

Interior of the House. There is a choice of patterns for the *ground-floor rooms*, all of which should open from the hall. A living room and kitchen are necessities, and the dining-room may be separate or combined with either, preferably as a recess big enough to accommodate the dining table, chairs, and either a built-in or movable sideboard to hold china, cutlery and table linen. Opening from the kitchen there may be a utility room or scullery, or the kitchen may be designed to include this. It is a very great benefit if there is an extra room, however small, for work or study.

The number of bedrooms must vary with the size of the family, and they will generally be on the first floor. Here also will be the bathroom which should not be combined with the water closet, unless on the ground floor there is a second water closet with a fixed lavatory basin.

Equipment and Fittings. Methods of *heating* will be according to individual choice, but in any case there should be arrangements for constant hot water. The projected plan of piping hot water from a central source to all houses in a given area may be a great benefit, but at present it is only in operation in certain blocks of flats. There is a wide variety of *cookers* and *water heaters* from which to choose, having regard to convenience and expense.

Electricity. This is easy and efficient, but expensive. There must be separate cookers and water heaters, each with thermostatic control. The water tank, which is fitted with an immersion heater, has to be "lagged" and there is no space heating to make the house warm and comfortable unless electric radiators are installed. The same disadvantages apply to the use of *gas* which, though suitable for cooking and water heating, is little used for space heating. There are various types of *modern insulated slow-combustion stoves* which are combined cookers and water heaters. Many models are recommended by The Coal Utilisation Council after research undertaken for The Ministry of Fuel and Power.

Larders should preferably face north, but this is not always possible, and *refrigerators* are very helpful for food storage; they are run by electricity or gas.

Cupboards should be built in, and should include store cupboards, a broom cupboard and a heated and ventilated linen cupboard. There should be provision for *clothes-washing* in the scullery or utility room, including a sink with a wringer, a boiler and hot drying rails. With regard to *sanitary fittings*, it is very desirable that cisterns fitted in the water closets should be types that flush quietly, and that lavatory pans should be self-cleansing. Pipes are placed as far as possible where they are protected, and those that are in exposed positions must be efficiently lagged. An omission in many otherwise well-designed modern houses, is *storage room* for trunks, chests and other necessities which cannot be kept in an outside shed. The essential *outbuildings* are a fuel shed and a storage shed for bicycles, tools, etc., both near the back entrance, and in most cases a garage.

Flats. These present special problems, the chief of which are noise, insufficient privacy and the absence of a private garden. There are difficulties too for families with young children, but for many people flats are the most convenient type of dwelling. Many blocks of flats have a grim and depressing appearance, but there is no need for this. The design and grouping of the blocks can be beautiful with varied levels of roof lines, balconies, courtyards and gardens.

Sound Insulation. It is of special importance to provide insulation against inside noise, and walls, and especially floors and ceilings, are designed to prevent sound transmission as far as possible. The use of thick carpets and underlays, or rubber carpets will reduce noise most effectively.

Balconies. These are a great asset, and should be private. Boxes and tubs of flowers give at least slight compensation for the absence of a private garden.

Lifts. There should be both passenger and service automatic lifts in every block of flats, as well as a staircase and sufficient outside fire-escape staircases.

Rooms. These should be as large as they would be in houses of a similar grade. Daylight in the rooms must be adequate. The higher the blocks of flats the wider should be the space between them. Blocks built in such shapes as Y or ⊓ are much better than the closed courtyard shape.

Heating. A system of central heating with electricity for separate units and cookers is the best method, because it disposes of the need for fuel storage. If there are open fireplaces there should be fuel storage facilities with outside approach. Hot water is best supplied to the flats by a central system.

Artificial Lighting. This may be by means of fluorescent strip lighting or separate lamps. There should be points for light, power and wireless in all rooms.

Refuse. Removal should be by means of chutes on each floor. They discharge into large bins which when full are closed and removed by the sanitary authorities, a fresh bin being left in exchange. In Leeds a system of water-borne refuse disposal has been tried in large blocks of flats. The kitchens have special sinks with wide-mouthed openings (hoppers) and large bore pipes. All refuse—tins, bottles, ashes, etc., is put in the hopper, water is turned on, a plunger is raised, and the refuse goes down the pipe which leads underground where the contents is carried by suction to a central chamber. Here the liquid flows into the sewer and the solids are passed into a furnace which heats water for the communal laundry. This method is practicable only for very large scale plans, owing to its cost, and a great disadvantage is the inevitable noise.

Laundry. Some blocks of flats are built with communal laundries, including washing, drying and ironing rooms. In others laundry equipment on a small scale is in the kitchen, and includes electrically heated drying rails which may be enclosed in a drying cabinet.

Storage. There should be provision on the ground floor for storing bicycles, perambulators, etc.

Garages. Plans should include a sufficient number of lock-up garages within easy access.

CHAPTER II

AIR AND VENTILATION

The Atmosphere

THE atmosphere is an envelope of gases surrounding the earth to a depth of 200 miles or more. Up to a height of seven miles it is known as the troposphere and above this the stratosphere. The composition of the atmosphere does not change on ascending, but it becomes rapidly more and more rarified. Temperature decreases on ascending up to a height of ten miles.

Composition of Air

			Per cent. of the volume.
Nitrogen	..	.. ..	79
Oxygen	..	.. ..	21 (nearly)
Carbon dioxide		.. ..	0·03
Argon, Hydrogen, Helium, etc.			Trace
Water vapour		.. ..	Very variable

Also in towns "smoke", by the sea salt crystals, and everywhere particles of "dust".

Oxygen is necessary for all combustion, inside and outside the body. It is roughly 21 per cent. of the atmosphere. On ascending, the air becomes rapidly less dense, until at a height of five miles there is not sufficient oxygen to sustain movement.

Carbon dioxide is produced by combustion inside the body and outside. The CO_2 in the air comes from:

1. The breathing of men and animals, as a result of tissue combustion.

2. The burning of all fuels.

1*

3. The breaking down of organic substances, plant and animal.

Plants need it, and breathe it in from the air, for the carbon it contains.

Its presence in the blood stimulates breathing and the body rids itself of excess in expired air.

Nitrogen has no action in animal life. It is not absorbed from the lungs, but is present in air, in which it dilutes the oxygen.

Argon is also inert.

Water vapour is present in the air from:

1. Evaporation from all water surfaces.
2. Evaporation from all moist surfaces, including skin, mucous membrane, leaves of plants, wet clothes, and the like.
3. Breath from the lungs of men and animals.

Pressure.

The weight or pressure of the air at sea level is about 14 lb. per square inch (1,000 millibars), but the pressure becomes rapidly less on ascending, since there is less weight of air above. As the pressure decreases the molecules of the gases are less densely pressed together and therefore the *volume* of the air increases.

Measuring Atmospheric Pressure.

The Barometer. It has been found that if a tube is filled with mercury, and inverted with the open end immersed in a bowl of mercury, the pressure of the atmosphere on the mercury in the bowl will keep the column of mercury standing in the tube *so long as the tube is not longer than 29–30 inches.* If it is longer the mercury will fall to the level of 29–30 inches (above the level of the mercury in the bowl), leaving a vacuum above. The pressure of atmosphere that will produce this result is found to be 14 lb. per square inch. When the atmospheric pressure becomes less, the mercury falls a little, and rises again when pressure increases. This is a very simple form of barometer.

Another type, the *aneroid barometer*, indicates the variations of air pressure by its effects on a thin corrugated metal box in which there is a partial vacuum. When air pressure falls the box expands, and as pressure rises it contracts. These changes are recorded by a pointer on a revolving drum marked in millibars.

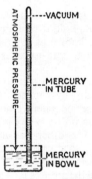

FIG. 2.—A SIMPLE BAROMETER.

Temperature.

The sun's rays travel through space and pass through the atmosphere without directly warming it, but warming the earth and water where they are absorbed. The air above these surfaces is warmed by contact and becoming lighter expands and rises, cooling gradually as it reaches high altitudes.

Thermometers used to measure air temperature are usually of the type containing a liquid (mercury or alcohol) that expands and contracts in a graduated glass tube. The Fahrenheit scale is used in some countries and Centigrade in others. Some thermometers (*e.g.* thermostats in ovens) operate by means of strips of metals that have different rates of expansion.

Humidity.

The amount of water vapour the air can hold depends upon its temperature. If the air at whatever temperature holds as much water vapour as it can it is said to be *saturated*. If its temperature increases it will take up more; if it cools some of the vapour will be condensed.

The ratio of the amount of water vapour in the air to the amount it would hold if saturated (the temperature being the same) is known as the *relative humidity*. If, for example, it could hold twice as much the relative humidity is 50 per cent.

Hygrometers are used in order to estimate humidity. A wet-and-dry-bulb hygrometer (or psychrometer) consists of two thermometers mounted side by side. One of these has an ordinary dry bulb and records the air temperature. The other has its bulb covered in muslin which dips into a little container of water below and so is always wet. Evaporation taking place from the wet muslin into the air uses heat and so the wet-bulb recording will be lower than the dry-bulb reading. These two readings used with a chart give the relative humidity.

Air Circulation.

Difference in density is responsible for movements of air whether on a large scale, as winds, or in small confined spaces, as in rooms. Temperature and moisture affect the density, or pressure, since (a) hot air expands, becoming lighter, and rises; and (b) moist air is less dense than dry air.

Convection currents, whether on a large scale, as winds, or on a small scale, in buildings, are caused by heated air rising, and cooler air from surrounding areas flowing in to take its place and, in its turn, becoming warm and rising.

Vertical currents may arise (often near mountains) when warm air rises, expands and cools and descending cool air becomes compressed and warmed. Such air currents cause *gusts* on a large scale, while, in towns, buildings cause gusts on a small scale by obstructing the steady flow of wind. One effect of this is felt indoors when a high gusty wind blowing over a chimney reduces the pressure in the top of the chimney so that air is sucked up from the room.

Large scale disturbance of the atmosphere is caused by areas of low pressure or *depressions* which move forward accompanied by areas of high pressure, the winds moving in spiral patterns towards the low pressure area.

POLLUTION OF AIR

The composition of the air may be changed, or impurities may be added, in various circumstances. The chief causes are:

1. Respiration.

The composition of air as expired is:

				Parts in every 100 *parts of Air.*
Oxygen	..	..	..	16
Nitrogen	..	..	..	79
Argon	..	..	..	1 (nearly)
Carbon dioxide	..	..	..	4·0
Water vapour	..	..	..	saturated.

Oxygen is reduced, but never low enough to cause discomfort under normal conditions, except in very crowded ill-ventilated rooms.

Carbon dioxide though increased in expired air, is harmless because it is immediately diluted on mixing with the atmosphere.

Water Vapour. Expired air is saturated. In a crowded, unventilated room the large amounts of moisture added to the air may cause discomfort.

Bacteria. In quiet breathing an invisible cloud of minute droplets is projected, it is said, to a distance of 5 feet, bearing large numbers of bacteria. In coughing and sneezing the spray of droplets may reach as far as 20 feet.

2. Combustion.

The most important and extensive cause of air pollution in Britain is incomplete combustion of fuels.

Complete combustion of all fuels produces the gases carbon dioxide, water vapour and sulphur dioxide.

Sulphur Gases. These are accountable for structural decay of historic buildings. They are comparatively heavy gases, and sulphur dioxide, rising from chimneys, combines with moisture in the air and forms sulphuric acid, which penetrates and disintegrates the stone. For this reason buildings are sprayed with a solution which prevents the crumbling of the stone.

Incomplete Combustion. This, in addition to the gases mentioned, adds to the atmosphere other products which are responsible for **atmospheric pollution.** The polluting substances vary with the type of fuel.

Coal when burned produces, in addition to the above gases, ash, clinker and grit, which passes up the chimney with the gases.

Gas, produced at the gas works is purified, so that the sulphur dioxide content is small.

Motor Spirit. In the exhaust gases (which are discharged at ground level) there is a high content of carbon monoxide. This gas if breathed in continuously or in high concentration is very poisonous because it combines with haemoglobin in the red blood cells in place of oxygen. (Carbon monoxide is present also in fumes from coke-burning closed stoves, so that care should be taken that there is no leak in the flue pipe.)

Diesel oil. Diesel engines are responsible for adding large quantities of sulphur dioxide to the atmosphere. If these are not in good condition they also pour out dense smoke at ground level.

Smoke.

This is produced as the result of incomplete combustion of coal and fuel oils. It consists of the gases carbon dioxide, water vapour and sulphur dioxide with solid particles of soot, fine dust and grit, and minute liquid droplets of tar and oil.

Smoke is discharged from: (a) domestic chimneys, (b) industrial chimneys, (c) chimneys of commercial premises, hospitals, etc., (d) railway engines and other transport sources.

The effects of smoke pollution are serious and costly as may be seen from the accompanying chart.

Methods of Prevention. These are the subject of intensive research, by a special department of the Fuel Research Board, and the following recommendations have been made for immediate adoption where possible.

(a) *Domestic Smoke.* This is discharged at low level and hangs over cities, reduces sunlight, induces fog, and causes ill health and also dirt and corrosion. There are various remedies under consideration.

(1) Prevention would be complete if there was exclusive use of smokeless fuel. This involves the replacing of old-fashioned grates by new models, and the provision of enough smokeless fuel for the whole country.

(2) Greater use of gas and electricity.

(3) The building of more blocks of flats with space

heating and hot water from central boilers. "District heating" for housing estates from single installations.

These are long-term remedies.

(b) *Industrial Smoke.* This is discharged from tall chimneys. It often contains a high concentration of sulphur dioxide. Recommendations are:

(1) The modernising of boiler-house equipment or the installation of new plant, particularly *mechanical stokers.*

(2) The extraction of grit from the flue gases of boilers by special apparatus.

(3) Training courses for boiler-house staff with special regard to the stoking of hand-fired boilers. It is now possible for stokers to obtain by examination a certificate issued by The City and Guilds of London Institute.

(c) *Transport.* Smoke could be greatly reduced by:

(1) Replacing shunting engines by diesel engines.
(2) Further electrification of railways.

Fog.

In certain circumstances these fogs become very dangerous to health as was seen in recent years when on one occasion London was blanketed under a thick yellow smoke fog (or "smog" as it was called) for some days, during which time the number of deaths in the metropolis was increased by several thousands and the hospitals were overcrowded by patients suffering from acute respiratory symptoms. It is believed that on this occasion the dangerous factor was the solution of sulphur dioxide in the moisture droplets forming round soot particles. The incomplete combustion of coal being the main cause. Some authorities have declared certain areas to be smokeless zones, in which under certain atmospheric conditions tending to

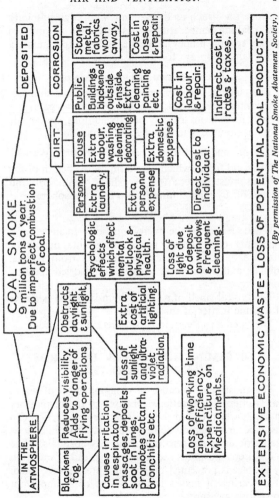

FIG. 3.—EFFECTS OF COAL SMOKE.

(By permission of The National Smoke Abatement Society.)

produce fog—such as little or no wind, high humidity and a falling temperature—it is forbidden to produce smoke from chimneys. Scientists are experimenting with chemical sprays for the dispersal of "smog".

3. Decomposition of Organic Matter.

This includes decaying vegetable matter and decomposing sewage, and the like. Offensive gases are given off but, under the best conditions, sewer air contains no more bacteria than does outside air.

4. Fumes and Dust from Chemical and Other Works.

Dust and fumes which would injure the health of the workers must be removed by exhaust ventilation and carried off by high chimneys into the atmosphere.

5. Dust.

When seen under the microscope, dust includes soot, fragments of material, pollen, fragments of plants, particles of rock, and organic particles from people, animals and insects, *e.g.* scales of skin, dried sputum, hairs, etc.

The typical smell of a stuffy room is due to particles of organic matter of this nature.

The open air after rain is considerably purified.

CONTAMINATION OF AIR IN WARDS AND SICKROOMS

The most serious cause of contamination of air in wards is **droplet infection.** Diseases of the respiratory passages are spread in this way and cross infection can easily occur. Haemolytic streptococcal throat infections are particularly dangerous in maternity hospitals, while in children's hospitals the danger of spread of infection by droplet is prevented only by the precautions taken. The wearing of masks is one of the most important preventive measures.

Dust is a potential source of infection in wards. In particular haemolytic streptococci and tubercle bacilli are very resistant to dehydration, and having been sprayed out in droplets by coughing, sneezing, etc., can remain alive in dust.

Care is taken in wards to avoid scattering dust. In modern wards construction is streamlined as far as possible, avoiding ledges and angled corners.

Furniture should be damp-dusted or polished and is frequently built-in.

Floors of all types should be cleaned first with suction sweepers. Rubber, stone and composite substances are then washed using a little disinfectant in the water, and for wood floors electric polishers are used.

Attention to cleanliness and good ventilation will keep the air fresh and pleasant.

VENTILATION

In a well ventilated room or building the air is fresh, at a comfortable temperature, and is constantly renewing and circulating. Freshness depends firstly on the outside surroundings. Open spaces, gardens and wide roads are the ideal environment in contrast to narrow sunless streets in crowded industrial areas. Inside a building freshness may be lost by the existence of any of the following conditions:

1. The presence of combustion products in the air from faulty heating units.
2. The smell from organic products on the skin and clothes of unwashed people or from nearby latrines.
3. Overheating.
4. Stagnation of the air.
5. In overcrowded, unventilated rooms the composition of the air changes gradually as oxygen is used up in breathing.

6. Bacteria and viruses are sprayed out by coughing and sneezing and infection is spread.

The effects of living and working in badly ventilated rooms are fatigue, lowered resistance to infection, irritability, and a lessened vitality. In schools and factories the "cooling power" of the air is tested, and must reach the required standard. This is specially important where much physical work is done. Muscle action produces heat which the body must lose through the skin, partly by radiation from the skin blood vessels, and partly by evaporation of sweat.

If the air is overheated, or there is excess moisture, and above all if it is stationary, this radiation and evaporation cannot take place and the result is a feeling of slackness and lethargy; the mind is dull, the body processes slow down, and there is a lowering of efficiency. In some cases suction ventilation is installed, and air conditioning plant may be added.

Laws about Air Space

In hospitals, factories, schools and other places where numbers of people live and work it is customary to regulate the air space per person occupying a room or ward.

Thus, with regard to hospitals, requirements are:
General ward: 1,400 cubic feet of air per bed.
Infectious ward: 2,000 cubic feet of air per bed.
(Height may not be reckoned more than 12 feet.)

In each case ventilation must be sufficient to change the air completely three times in an hour.

In infectious wards each bed must have 12 feet of wall space.

In actual practice the spacing of beds is strictly observed but, as regards ventilation, the changing of air three times an hour is the "letter of the law", the spirit of the law being observed by *continuous* changing of the air far in excess of regulations. In these days wards are often built with whole sides that can be thrown open to the air when weather is suitable.

Recent laws with regard to overcrowding (Housing Act of 1935, now consolidated in Housing Act of 1936) base the regulations on *floor space* instead of cubic space. Thus, where the floor area of a room is:

    (*a*) 110 square feet: 2 persons are allowed.
    (*b*) 70–90 square feet: 1 person is allowed.
    (*c*) Under 50 square feet: Nil.

(Children under one year are not taken into account, and from one to ten years are considered as half a unit.)

Methods of Ventilation

In the outside world the air is washed by *rain*, purified by *sunlight*, and ventilated by *winds* and *air currents*.

Over large areas of land or water air that is heated rises, and cooler heavier air from some adjacent area flows in to take its place. Even if the air is not felt to be moving, *diffusion* is taking place continuously.

Just as gas from a leaking gas pipe diffuses quickly through the air of a room, so do masses of air of different density (due to temperature or moisture) diffuse until the whole mass of air is of the same density.

Ventilation of Buildings and Rooms.

There are two types of ventilation:

    1. Natural, making use of the normal movements of air.
    2. Artificial, when air is forced through a building or sucked out from it.

Natural Ventilation of Rooms. This takes place by means of windows, doors, ventilators and fireplaces, if these are present.

The natural forces act in the following ways:

1. Through open windows—the wind blows in. This is called *perflation*.

2. The wind blowing across a chimney, causes a lowering of pressure in the top of it and thus sucks up air from the room below. This is *aspiration*. It is much more intense if there is a fire in the grate, because heated air always rises.

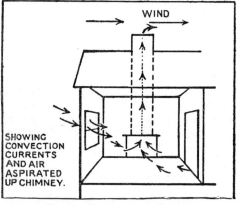

FIG. 4.—CONVECTION CURRENTS.

3. Heat from a fire, radiator, etc., striking on a surface, warms that surface. The heat from the surface warms the air immediately in contact with it, which thus becomes lighter and rises, while colder air flows in to take its place. This flowing of heated air is known as *convection currents*.

4. The "natural" ventilation of a room heated by central heating, and with no fireplace, is as follows: the air which enters through windows, doors, or special inlets, circulates round the heated pipes and radiators,

rises, and some of it passes out through perforated
bricks or gratings high up in the walls, or through open
window tops.   In this way convection currents are set
up, but they are less effectual than air currents in a room
with a chimney.   The windows may act as inlets, outlets, or, if open top and bottom, as both.

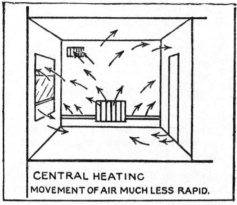

CENTRAL HEATING
MOVEMENT OF AIR MUCH LESS RAPID.

FIG. 5.—VENTILATION OF A ROOM WITH CENTRAL HEATING.

It is advisable that:

(a) Outlets should be high in the wall, since the
    heated (and contaminated) air rises.
(b) Inlets should be lower, but not on floor level,
    or there will be a cold draught across the
    floor.
(c) Inlets and outlets should not be exactly opposite
    each other, or the air simply crosses without
    circulating.

5. *Cross ventilation* may be useful in a patient's room.
His window is open (much or little).   The door is open,

and screened from his view, and windows of rooms on the opposite side of the corridor are opened, so causing a current of air right through.

Helps to Natural Ventilation. Certain mechanical structures have been devised to help ventilation. They are inserted in walls or windows to provide an inlet for air, when for some reason windows cannot be open, or further inlets are needed. They are:

> Extraction and intake fans.
> Hopper sashes.
> Tobin's tubes.
> Cooper's discs.
> Louvred panes.
> Perforated bricks and gratings.
> Sherringham valves.
> Various types of roof ventilators.
> Arnott's valve with mica flap for drains.
> Hinckes-Bird method for sash windows.
> (See Figs. 6–8.)

In rooms that are difficult to ventilate the most useful and efficient method of ensuring good air conditions is by the fitting of **Ventaxia** units in the walls or windows. These are worked by an electric motor and can be switched on and off as desired. They may be fitted for *extraction of stale air* or *intake of fresh air* and are of special value in steamy kitchens, classrooms, offices and basements. This is in effect mechanical ventilation on a small scale.

Mechanical Ventilation. In all large buildings and in places where steam, fumes and dust are present, mechanical ventilation is necessary. Air (sometimes heated) may be drawn in and blown through ducts into the building; this is the **Plenum System.** Alternatively, air may be sucked out through ducts by powerful extraction fans and passed into the atmosphere; this is the **Extraction System.**

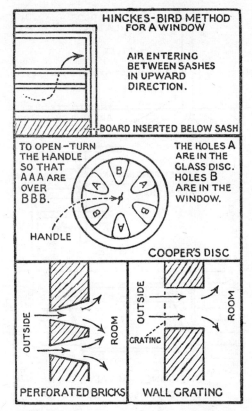

HINCKES-BIRD METHOD FOR A WINDOW

AIR ENTERING BETWEEN SASHES IN UPWARD DIRECTION.

BOARD INSERTED BELOW SASH

TO OPEN—TURN THE HANDLE SO THAT A A A ARE OVER B B B.

THE HOLES A ARE IN THE GLASS DISC. HOLES B ARE IN THE WINDOW.

HANDLE

COOPER'S DISC

OUTSIDE ROOM

PERFORATED BRICKS

OUTSIDE ROOM GRATING

WALL GRATING

FIG. 6.—HELPS TO NATURAL VENTILATION.

When the two methods are combined, as often they are, it is known as the **Balance System.** Such premises as theatres, cinemas, large kitchens, restaurants, factories and workshops, laboratories, ships and all other

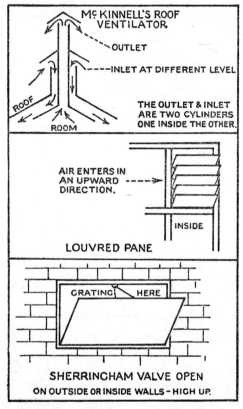

FIG. 7.—HELPS TO NATURAL VENTILATION.

very large buildings can be ventilated only by this means.

In factories where fumes and dust are produced the mechanical methods of ventilation that are used are

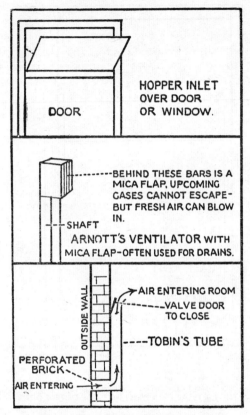

FIG. 8.—HELPS TO NATURAL VENTILATION.

very specialised as, for instance, in paint-spraying workshops where fume removal is combined with drying.

Testing the Efficiency of the Ventilation of Large Rooms and Buildings. The cooling power of the air of

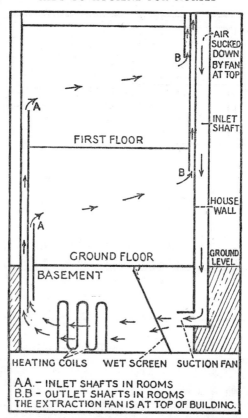

FIG. 9.—DIAGRAM ILLUSTRATING PRINCIPLE OF MECHANICAL VENTILATION.

a room is discovered by using the *Kata Thermometer*. Note is made of the time taken for the temperature to fall a certain number of degrees, first with the bulb dry, and then wrapped in wet muslin. The air of the room brings about this fall of temperature, and if this air does not dry the wet muslin and cool the thermometer quickly, it will not evaporate sweat from the skin and keep the workers sufficiently cool.

Air Conditioning

Methods of controlling air condition have been developed rapidly, and air-conditioning plants, either complex or simple, are now frequently installed. Three processes are involved:

(1) The air is filtered by being passed through a screen which removes dust and dirt;
(2) The air is humidified to a comfortable degree;
(3) The temperature is controlled by circulating the air over hot pipes in cold weather, or cold brine-filled pipes in warm weather.

Air that is treated in this way, cleaned, humidified, and warmed or cooled as required, can thus be made available in any building. Such plants are now installed in new operating theatres in order to prevent dust infection of operation wounds with sporing bacilli. Very highly specialised air-conditioning plants are installed in research laboratories capable of producing tropical or arctic climates.

CHAPTER III

HEATING AND LIGHTING

The Nature of Heat and Light

STUDENTS may wish to approach the practical application of heating and lighting by consideration of the nature of heat and light. The following is a simplified description of the structure of the atom and of the changes that take place in it resulting in the production of radiations.

The Structure of the Atom

All matter is composed of *elements* of which 92 different kinds are found in nature. The smallest unit of which an element is composed is an *atom*. The *atom* itself, however, has now been found to be composed of smaller particles of which the most important are *electrons*, *protons* and *neutrons*. These small particles in different numbers and arrangements make up the different atoms of the elements.

It is now believed that an atom consists of a central nucleus with electrons circulating round the nucleus in orbits just as the planets circulate round the sun. The nucleus itself consists of protons and neutrons and is positively charged. The neutrons carry no electric charge.

The positively charged protons are neutralized by negatively charged electrons circulating in the orbital rings, so that the atom remains electrically neutral.

The orbits or "shells" in which electrons circulate represent levels of energy. If an element is heated the energy of the atom is increased, the electrons moving to a shell of greater energy, and when they move back to their former level they will give out this energy. *Energy escapes the atom in the form of alpha and beta particles, infra-red rays, visible light, ultra-violet light, and gamma rays.*

In stable elements there is a definite ratio between the numbers of protons and neutrons in the nucleus, and if changes take place in this ratio the element becomes unstable or radio-active. Radio-active decay is the name given to the change occurring in an unstable atomic nucleus. The decay is always at a constant rate which is usually expressed by means of its half-life— the time taken for the activity of a given quantity to decay to half its initial value. In the case of radium the half-life is 1,590 years, in the case of iodine $8 \cdot 0$ days, and in the case of polonium less than one-millionth of a second.

The process of radio-active decay in elements produces varieties of the element known as **Isotopes.** (Some isotopes are radio-active while others are stable.) The radio-active isotopes are sometimes used in medicine, as for example radio-active iodine for cancer of the thyroid gland. Radio-active cobalt as a substitute for radium, etc.

Electromagnetic waves produced by energy streaming out from disturbed atoms vary in wave length depending on the nature of the atoms (carbon, radium, etc.).

The wave length is the measurement from crest to crest thus:

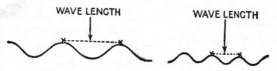

FIG. 10.—MEASUREMENT OF WAVE LENGTH.

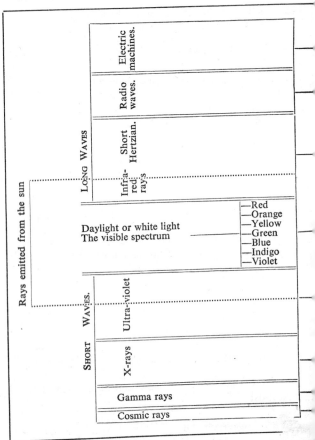

FIG. 11.—DIAGRAM TO SHOW THE

$\longrightarrow$ { Used in diathermy to produce heat in deep tissues and in electrical treatments.

$\longrightarrow$ { Very long waves measured in metres; used in wireless transmission.

$\longrightarrow$ { Invisible rays.
They penetrate the surface layer of skin and are absorbed in the deeper layer, producing heat.

$\longrightarrow$ { Visible rays, because they are absorbed by the retina of the eye.

$\longrightarrow$ { Invisible rays.
They are absorbed by the upper layer of the skin and produce tanning.
They produce vitamin D in the skin.
They kill bacteria on the surface.
They stimulate metabolism.

$\longrightarrow$ { They penetrate through many substances, but are absorbed by bone, metal, barium salts and other substances, so are used to throw shadows on prepared films and screens.
They kill cancer cells.

$\longrightarrow$ { From radium.
They kill cancer cells.

$\longrightarrow$ The shortest rays known at present.

VARIOUS WAVE LENGTHS (not to scale).

2

The very long ones, *e.g.* radio waves, are measured in metres, while the very short, such as radium, are measured by a unit which is a ten-millionth part of a millimetre.

Waves or rays travel in straight lines from their source, and when they reach objects in their path they produce effects which depend on how the object *absorbs* them, and this in turn depends on the wave length.

Wireless waves which are long travel silently until they are absorbed by a receiver which converts them into sound.

Certain long rays are absorbed by the skin where they affect the nerve endings and are felt as heat; these are the *infra-red* rays. Still longer ones pass right through the skin to be absorbed by, and produce heat in, deeper tissues. These are *diathermy* rays.

Ultra-violet rays, which are short waves, are absorbed by the upper layer of the skin and produce sunburn.

Between the infra-red and the ultra-violet is a band of *visible* (*light*) *rays* which are absorbed by the retina of the eye.

Still others, *X-rays*, penetrate all the less dense substances and are absorbed by bone and metal.

HEAT

Heat rays from the sun, after passing through the atmosphere, reach the surface of the earth where they are absorbed, producing warmth. This process of *radiation* has very little effect on the air, which is heated by contact with the warm earth, the warmed air rising and giving place to cooler air which is warmed in its turn. This process is heating by *convection*. The soil is warmed below the surface by heat passing from particles to other particles in contact, *i.e.* heating by *conduction*.

Transmission of Heat. These examples from nature illustrate the three methods by which heat is transmitted:

> Radiation.
> Convection.
> Conduction.

Radiation. Heat rays stream out from any body heated to a high temperature, *e.g.* from the sun, or from coal or wood if combustion is taking place, from a heated metal reflector behind an electric coil, and the like. These heat rays travel in straight lines, having little effect on the air as they pass through, but heating the people or objects on which they strike. (The *air* of the room is warmed by contact with the heated walls, furniture, etc., and circulates, heating by convection.) The people in the front ring round a fire are heated by radiation, but others, on whom the rays do not strike, are warmed by the air.

Radiated heat rapidly loses its intensity with distance, so that the far end of a large room heated by a fire may be comparatively cold.

Examples of heating by radiation are the sun, coal and wood fires, gas fires, electric fires.

Convection. This is the method by which air and liquids are heated.

(*a*) *Air.* Some heated object such as a hot pipe or stove warms the air next to it. This air, being light, rises, and cooler air flows in to take its place. This, in turn, is heated and rises, and the process continues, the air of the room circulating and becoming continually warmer.

(b) *Liquids.* The process is the same, heated liquid rising and cooler sinking on to the heated surface of

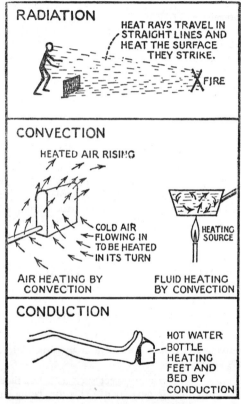

FIG. 12.—METHOD OF HEATING.

the kettle or pan, where it in turn becomes hot and rises, so circulating continually until it boils.

In both these cases the molecules of air and water actually move, rising, circulating and sinking continuously.

Conduction. A hot object is in contact with a cool one—*e.g.*, a fire with a poker, or a hot-water bottle with a person or sheets. Heat passes from the hot object to the cool one and on through it, each particle heating the next, till the whole object is hot. Some substances conduct heat much better than others, and therefore quickly become hot. Examples are:

Good conductors: All metals, mercury.

Bad conductors: Water, air, wood, paper.

Heating the House

The best method of obtaining a comfortable temperature and a good supply of hot water in the many new houses under construction has been the subject of much research undertaken for the Ministry of Fuel and Power. Important reports have been made on fuels, heating appliances and insulation of houses, and both Local Authorities and private builders are concerned to reach the standards recommended. Pre-war houses outnumber new ones by at least ten to one, and it is possible though more difficult, to improve heating efficiency in these.

Modern standards aim at maintaining a temperature of 45° to 50° F. through the whole house, which is termed "*background heating*". This should be supplemented by separate units in each room for "topping up", that is increasing the temperature to about 65° F. in the living room and 55° F. in bedrooms. Hot water at about 140° F. should be laid on to baths, basins and sinks.

In putting these recommendations into practice, there are three subjects to consider:

(1) Insulation (of new houses).

(2) Appliances for background heating and hot water supply.

(3) Separate heating units for providing extra warmth.

1. Insulation.   The purpose is to prevent the considerable heat loss through walls, floors and roofs.

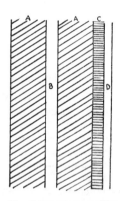

Fig. 13.—Insulation of Walls.
(A) Brickwork 44 in.; (B) 2 in. cavity; (C) 11 in. woodwork; (D) Plaster.

External Walls.   The usual type of brick wall with a 2 inch cavity may be lined on its inner side under the plaster finish with a "blanket" of wood wool.

Floors.   Under the floor is a ventilated space, and over the joints but below the floor boards there may be laid a draped "quilt" of wood wool. Alternatively, a wood block floor may be laid in bitumen on a concrete foundation.

Roofs. Over the ceiling joists a "quilt" of wood wool or glass silk may be draped.

The effect of this type of construction is to double the efficiency of the heating system and therefore reduce the consumption of fuel. These standards of insulation in new houses are not at present obligatory, but they are officially recommended.

2. Background Heating. Modern systems heat the house by means of hot water pipes and radiators, or by

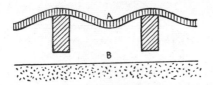

FIG. 14.—FLOOR INSULATION.

(A) 1 in. silk or slag wool quilt draped over joists; (B) Ventilated under-floor space.

ducted hot air. The heating unit may burn solid smokeless fuel (anthracite, phurnacite or coke) oil, or gas. Solid fuel units may be openable, giving extra heat by radiation. Oil-fired units are automatic and thermostatically controlled. If the heating is by ducted air, the warm air passes up ducts in the walls and enters the rooms through grilles. Combined with space-heating, the unit usually provides the hot water supply for the whole house. The boiler connects with a storage tank (which should be in the airing cupboard) from which hot water is distributed to baths, sinks, etc.

Lagging of Tanks and Pipes. Hot water tanks should be lagged even though they are intended to heat the linen cupboard. This will greatly reduce the heat-loss and so save fuel. Cold water pipes if exposed to cold air and draughts should be lagged to avoid the nuisance

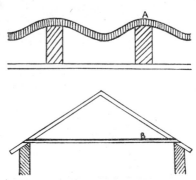

FIG. 15.—ROOF INSULATION.

(A) 1 in. glass silk or slag wool quilt draped over joists;
(B) Position of insulating quilt.

of frozen pipes. Some of the flexible materials used for lagging tanks and pipes are: asbestos, glass wool, slag wool, compressed felt. They are made up in the form of quilts or strips, or ready-to-fit jackets for tanks.

3. Separate Heating Units. These are used to provide extra heat in rooms. They may be open fires, gas fires or electric heaters.

Open Fires.

The modern models are very different from older types; they give out much more heat for little more than half the quantity of fuel. Many burn continuously day and night, having an adjustable air control to regulate the rate of burning. Smokeless fuels may be used—coke, anthracite, etc., or, if preferred, household coal. They are inset, being fixed into existing fireplace openings. Some have a hinged closure lid which can be adjusted to reduce the rate of burning at night to the minimum needed to keep the fire alight.

The "*convector*" open fire is a modern type which, in addition to the heat radiated from the fire, provides warm air convected through grilles into the room. Behind the grate is an air space into which cool air enters either under or above the floor; there it is heated, and then passes out into the room through a grille above the fireplace, thus greatly increasing the efficiency of the grate. The warmed air may also be passed by a duct into the room above.

Both types of open grate may have a built-in back boiler for hot water supply, or may be combined with cookers.

The *position of the chimney stack* should be on an inside wall, so that heat will not be "lost up the chimney" but, by heating the brickwork, will help to warm adjacent rooms.

The *design* of the grate is planned to improve heating efficiency by means of a narrow chimney throat, a forward-sloping fireclay back, and a wide front to increase radiation.

Smokeless Fuel. The importance of the use of smokeless fuels for domestic fires cannot be overestimated in the campaign for reducing fog.

Gas Fires.

Gas used for heating is normally produced from coal, but may be produced by combustion of other substances. The three primary products resulting from

2*

distillation of coal are: raw coal gas, coal tar, and coke. From these an enormous number of by-products is obtained, including many of the most useful disinfectants. The accompanying chart shows some of these and also the composition of purified coal gas, and the origin of some of the various fuels obtained from coal.

Gas fires consist of a number of "fuels" made of fireclay placed against a fireclay back. Gas points at the base heat these and the heat is radiated as from coal fires, the air being warmed by convection from heated walls and furniture. Some models stand on a tiled hearth, and others are built in, set in coloured panels. They are clean, labour saving and convenient. Flueless portable gas fires are often used (and also flueless cookers) but ventilation needs to be efficient since the products of combustion are discharged into the room.

Gas cookers and *ranges, dishwashing machines* and all kinds of gas catering equipment are much used.

Gas water heaters are separate appliances either of the "geyser" type or with a storage tank, and may be single or multi-point.

Gas is measured in *British Thermal Units* (B.Th.U.).

A "*B.Th.U.*" is the amount of heat required to raise the temperature of 1 lb. of water through 1° F.

A *therm* is 100,000 B.Th.U.'s, and 1 therm is 200 cubic feet of gas. The cost varies, but gas is always more expensive than solid fuel.

Oil.

Paraffin oil is extremely useful for heating on a small or large scale. Oil-fired central heating appliances are easy to manage and efficient, whether in large buildings or in houses.

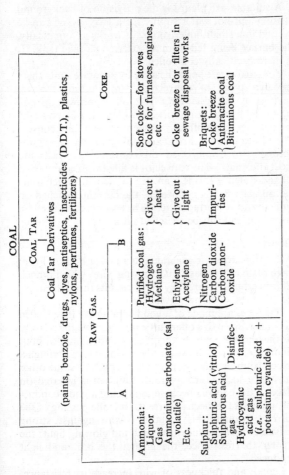

COAL

COAL TAR

Coal Tar Derivatives
(paints, benzole, drugs, dyes, antiseptics, insecticides (D.D.T.), plastics, nylons, perfumes, fertilizers)

RAW GAS.

A

Ammonia:
Liquor
Gas
Ammonium carbonate (sal volatile)
Etc.

Sulphur:
Sulphuric acid (vitriol)
Sulphurous acid } Disinfec-
gas } tants
Hydrocyanic acid gas +
(i.e. sulphuric acid + potassium cyanide)

B

Purified coal gas:
Hydrogen } Give out
Methane } heat
Ethylene } Give out
Acetylene } light
Nitrogen } Impuri-
Carbon dioxide } ties
Carbon mon-oxide

COKE.

Soft coke—for stoves
Coke for furnaces, engines, etc.

Coke breeze for filters in sewage disposal works

Briquets:
Coke breeze
Anthracite coal
Bituminous coal

FIG. 16.—DIAGRAM TO SHOW SOME OF THE PRODUCTS OF DISTILLATION OF COAL.

A suitable size plant for the provision of background heating and hot water supply for a large house can be housed in a small boiler room. It works automatically, the burner being fed from an external storage tank. It is thermostatically controlled.

For small scale space heating by separate units there are two types of convectors. (*a*) Portable heaters having an oil reservoir. The oil is drawn up and vaporised by the heat, burning with a blue flame as the vapour is mixed with air. Open grilles allow convection of heated air. Frequent refilling of the reservoir is needed. (*b*) Compressed oil convectors. These are most effectual. The convector is filled with compressed oil and sealed. Inside is an electric element which heats the oil. The flex is connected, the current switched on and control is thermostatic. These convectors need no attention, and can be switched off at will.

Electricity.

Electric current is generated in a power house. From there main cables pass out, carrying wires which branch off into houses, where they make circuits through lamps, electric fires, cooking stoves, etc.

The wires are made of a good conducting metal, such as copper, since this offers little resistance to the passage of the current, which therefore flows along without hindrance. When, however, the wiring passes through a fire or lamp or other apparatus, a length of some other substance such as iron wire or tungsten is inserted (in place of the copper) because, not being a good conductor, it resists the electric current. It is the passing of the current through this length of wire against strong resistance that produces the heat and glowing light; the greater the resistance, the greater heat and light produced.

Length and thickness of wire increase its resistance, so it is usually closely coiled, in order to make it as long as possible. When the circuit of the wire is broken the current ceases to pass: it is "switched off".

Short Circuits. Should some obstruction occur in the wiring, or should the current be too strong, the wire would be overheated and would melt, and possibly set fire to anything inflammable near it. The circuit would of course be broken, but the current, not being cut off, would pass on through anything in contact with the wire, hence the danger of touching it.

Fuses are used in order to prevent this. A fuse is a short piece of some metal that melts at a fairly low temperature. It is inserted in the circuit, and if the wire becomes heated the fuse melts and breaks the circuit. In order to prevent the current short-circuiting, fuse wires are placed in fireproof cases and insulated from the wall by porcelain.

Measurement. Electricity is measured in kilowatts. One kilowatt is 1000 watts. The amount of energy or power consumed is reckoned in kilowatt-hours and one kilowatt-hour is expressed as one unit.

Wiring. A new system of wiring has recently been introduced known as the "Ring Main". Instead of many pairs of wires radiating from the main fuse board to all plug points the new system provides a single pair of wires coming from the meter end and returning there after feeding all the plug points in the house. Each plug point can be used for any purpose—lighting, heating, radio, etc., the maximum current that can be taken from one plug point being 3 kilowatts (a 3-bar electric fire). There is a fuse in the top of each plug point. By this means a faulty appliance will blow *only* its own fuse.

Heating by Electricity. As a means of heating by *separate units*, electric fires have particular advantages. They are clean, labour saving, portable if desired and, since there is no combustion, there are no harmful products requiring a flue for removal. Space heating by electricity is also a useful method, but is not at present widely used owing to shortage of generating plant.

Electric Fires. (1) *The fire-bar type.* This has 1, 2 or 3 bars (coils) backed by fireclay and mounted in many designs. Most of the heat output is by radiation, but there is also a large percentage of convected heat by means of openings at the top or back through which warmed air rises into the room.

(2) *The reflector type.* The heating element is closely coiled on a fireclay rod which is mounted on a polished metal bowl or other shape. Most of the heat is given off as a beam of radiant heat.

Background Heating. This is by means of convectors, radiant panel heaters, or electric radiators.

(*a*) *Convectors* or *tubular heaters.* These are low temperature heaters. The tubes heat up to about 180° F. and are useful installed round skirtings. Other types of convectors are in the form of cabinets for drying and airing. These contain an element which warms the air to a moderate temperature. The air enters at floor level and passes out at the top of the cabinet.

(*b*) *Radiant heaters.* These are metal panels enclosing heating elements and backed with insulating material. They are fixed to walls or may be free-standing and portable. They are thermostatically controlled.

Electric Water Heating. There are two methods available. An immersion heater may be fitted into a storage tank or, alternatively, an electric water heater of about $1\frac{1}{2}$ to 3 gallons capacity can be fixed over the sink. In both cases there is thermostatic control.

Central Heating or Space Heating on a Large Scale

There are four methods of central heating in common use today:

1. **Low-Pressure System.** Water circulates at a temperature of about 180° F. in pipes 3 inches in diameter.

2. **High-Pressure System.** The pipes are much smaller in diameter ($\frac{7}{8}$ inch), and they pass in coils *through* the furnace so that the water is heated to a temperature much above boiling-point. The air in the building is liable to be overheated.

3. **Steam Heating.** Steam circulates through the pipes. This method greatly overheats the air.

4. **Panel Heating.** The heating units are panels, let into the walls or ceilings, and the heating of the panels is by hot water pipes or electricity. They may be painted over, and being flush with the wall and ceiling they are not at all conspicuous. The heating is by radiation on to the floors or furniture, and these heat the air by convection. Each unit is separately controlled by a switch or tap, and so temperature can be regulated.

Description of a Low-Pressure System as adapted to a Hospital.

In a furnace house there is a furnace surrounded by a boiler from which *steam* passes out by a pipe at the top (pipe A in Fig. 17), which branches to all the buildings and departments.

In each building the steam pipe passes into a *calorifier*, that is, a tank of water in which the pipe forms a *coil* which heats the water.

Circulation of the Water. From the calorifier, water at a temperature of about 180° F. passes out by a pipe at the top (pipe B) and circulates through pipes and radiators in rooms, wards and corridors, returning to the calorifier for reheating.

Return of the Steam to the Boiler. The steam-pipe (A), after forming the coil in the calorifier, leads to—

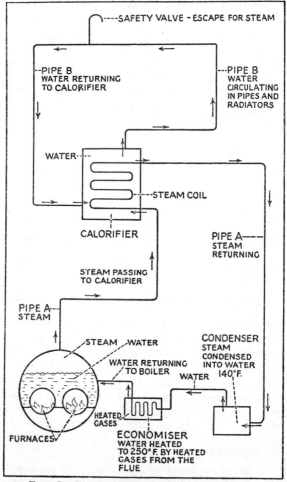

FIG. 7.—DIAGRAM SHOWING METHOD OF CENTRAL HEATING BY A LOW-PRESSURE SYSTEM.

The condenser, where the steam is condensed into water. From there, on its way to the boiler, it is pumped through—

The economizer, an apparatus in the flue, between the boiler and the chimney. In it the water flows through a number of cast-iron pipes, surrounded by greatly heated waste gases from the furnace. The water arriving in the economizer at a temperature of perhaps 140° F. is heated by these gases to a temperature much above boiling-point. (Soot that collects on the pipes is removed by "scrapers" or "blowers".) From here the water returns to—

The boiler, where it is again converted into steam, much less fuel being required for this than would be the case if the water had not been heated in the economizer.

There are many calorifiers in the course of a big system, some for the heating pipes, others for bath water and others for kitchen use. There are also coils in the sterilizers of theatres and wards.

Heating is by convection three times repeated: (1) Water in the furnace boiler heats by convection; (2) water in the calorifiers heats and circulates by convection; and (3) the air in the rooms is heated from pipes and radiators by convection.

Safety valves are placed in the top pipes of the heating system to make a way of escape for steam if the water boils. The pressure of the steam forces them open.

The Heating Coils in Rooms, Wards and Corridors. The coils of pipes that heat the rooms may be installed in various positions and designs.

Visible. The heating surface of the pipes is supplemented by radiators, which are coils of pipes, raised from the floor, painted in suitable colours and controlled by valves. The name "radiator" is misleading, as air is always heated by convection.

Invisible. This is the newest method. There are no visible pipes, and therefore nothing to collect dust or interfere with decoration schemes. There are two systems in use.

(*a*) *Panel System.* Metal panels are inserted in the wall, and heated by pipe coils behind them. The panels heat the air of the room, and each pipe coil is controlled separately by a valve. (In some cases the panels are electrically heated and controlled by switches.)

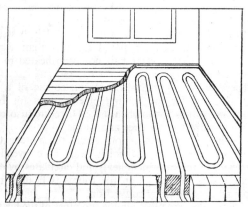

FIG. 18.—"PANELITE" FLOOR HEATING.
It may be applied to walls or ceilings in the same way.

(*b*) *The "Panelite" System.* In this system the pipe coils are built into the ceiling, walls, or floor of a room. They are laid over the whole surface, behind the plaster or concrete, or under the floor blocks, and each pipe is encased in a special covering to prevent any risk in case of overheating of the water. The heating is very even, and the system is often chosen for modern buildings, especially hospitals.

Points with Regard to Central Heating.

1. Ventilation is not helped. Perforated bricks, gratings and other devices are built into walls to remedy this defect as far as possible.

2. The air may become overheated and lack freshness, but open windows and efficient control of steam to the calorifiers should prevent this.

3. It makes no dirt or labour, but walls and ceilings are discoloured where hot pipes run if they are left exposed.

Heating of Hospitals.

Central heating is often supplemented by electric or coal fires for the benefit of convalescent patients and the staff.

Panel heating, by hot water or electricity, and the concealed pipes system are the most modern methods.

LIGHTING

Light is the sensation produced when rays of certain wave lengths reach the eye and are absorbed by the retina. These rays travel out from their source at a speed of 186,000 miles (300 million metres) per second.

Daylight is the white light produced by the combined seven wave lengths that comprise the visible rays from the sun and which, seen separately, are the seven colours of the spectrum.

Colour. The substances and materials of which different objects are made often do not absorb all the seven colour waves. When a ray of light falls on some object, whichever rays it does not absorb are reflected back, and strike the retina of the eye, so that we "see" the *reflected* colour (and not those colours that are absorbed).

For example, light falls on grass, and all the colour rays are absorbed by it except the green rays. These

are reflected back on to the retina of the eye, and we
see "green". This happens whenever we look at grass
so we say that grass is green. Again, in looking at red
poppies, the petals do not absorb the red rays, so they
are thrown back on to our eyes, and we see red. We
therefore say the poppies are red.

If all the seven colour rays are absorbed, none are
reflected back to our eyes, and we say the object is
black. If none of the rays are absorbed, the whole beam
of light is reflected back, and we say the object is white.

Glass lets through the rays of the visible spectrum
and some of the infra-red rays, but not the ultra-violet
rays (except in the case of vita glass). To make
coloured glass, some substance must be put into it
which will absorb all the colour rays except the colour
desired, so that those rays only will pass through and
reach the eye, and the glass will appear to be that colour.

Natural Lighting

In private houses windows usually form at least one-
third of the area of the walls of the house. The modern
tendency in hospitals is to construct wards with as much
window space as possible. Windows are made to
extend as nearly from floor to ceiling as is practicable,
and in some cases the whole side of a ward can be
thrown open by means of folding and sliding windows.
Ultra-violet rays, with their power of killing bacteria
and improving metabolism, do not penetrate through
ordinary glass, but *vita glass*, which is sometimes used,
transmits them.

Some Types of Windows.

Sash windows.

Casement windows, with the upper part a hopper sash.

Pivot windows.—The whole window swings round on
a central rod. They can be adapted to the wind, and
are easy to clean.

Folding and sliding windows which enable large areas, or the whole side of a ward, to be thrown open.

Louvred windows. The whole window consists of three or four louvred panes.

Where rooms face on to a noisy street, double windows may be fitted, but some type of ventilator is then necessary.

Reflecting surfaces greatly affect the lighting of rooms, and wall colourings are important in hospitals. Greens and blues in pastel shades are restful, and cream is nearly always pleasing.

If it is necessary to use rooms the windows of which look on to a close wall, the wall should be whitewashed.

Artificial Lighting

Measurement of Light. Lighting is gauged in foot-candles. One foot-candle is the light received at a point one foot distant from a source of light of one candle-power (C.P.). A gas-filled 60 watt lamp is equal to about 46 C.P. and a 100 watt lamp to 92 C.P.

The points to be considered in arranging lighting of rooms, wards, etc., are:

(*a*) The power of the light.

(*b*) Type of lighting, which may be:

1. Direct: Light is thrown *down* by an over-shade. (Glare may be prevented by using pearl or frosted bulbs.)

2. Indirect: Light is thrown *up* by an under-shade on to the ceiling, which reflects it down.

3. Semi-indirect: Some light passes through a diffusing bowl, and some is reflected from the ceiling.

4. Diffused: The light is totally enclosed in a diffusing glass bowl and the result is both direct and reflected light.

(c) Reflecting surfaces: The amount of light reflected depends on:

1. The colour of walls and ceiling.
2. The surface of walls and ceiling.
3. The cleanliness of walls and ceiling.

The following are in order of reflecting power:

Colour.	*Surface.*
White.	Mirrors.
Cream.	White tiles.
Yellow.	White paint.
Buff.	Aluminium and chromium plate.
Pink.	Light stone.
Light green.	Clean red brick.
Grey.	Dirty light paint.
Sky blue.	Dirty stone.
Green.	Dirty red brick.
Brown.	
Crimson.	

Electric Lighting.

There are two methods in use: filament lamps and fluorescent tubes, or strip lighting.

Lamps are filled with argon (since it is an inert gas) and a fine tungsten filament is inserted, which offers a high resistance to the current passing through, and so becomes intensely luminous. The filament may be a single-coil or a coiled-coil, which gives more light but also more glare, and needs good shading. Lamps may be clear, pearl, or silica-coated, and the wattage varies between 15 W. and 150 W.

Filament lamps are also made in tubular shape, the tubes being from 12 to 22 inches long.

The arrangement of the shades makes the lighting direct, reflected down from the ceiling, or diffused, and should be so managed as to avoid glare.

Fluorescent lighting compared with tungsten filament

lamps uses less power, gives a stronger light, casts no shadow, and causes no glare.

Vapour filled tubes are coated inside with fluorescent powders of various colours. When current is passed through, ultra-violet rays act on the fluorescent substances and brilliant coloured light is produced. Standard 5 foot tubes are much used, but 2, 3 or 4 foot tubes are also made. The light is well diffused and ideal for desk work, restaurants, shops, and all large rooms. The tubes may be fixed in "channels", or fitted with white enamelled reflectors or perspex diffusers, and they may be attached to the ceiling, or suspended. They are made in white, soft-tone, daylight, and various colours.

Artificial Lighting in Hospitals. *Wards.* Good general lighting is necessary, and is usually obtained by big central lights with translucent shades. It is greatly helped by reflected light from light-coloured glossy walls. In addition, local lights are needed, *e.g.* over beds, desks, etc. and, if either the shade or the lamp itself is adjustable, it will greatly add to the patient's comfort. At night blue bulbs are sometimes put up in place of white ones over beds where light is needed or, alternatively, a method of dimming may be in use.

Corridors. General lighting may be by shaded lights as for wards, or any of the built-in methods. Signal lamps, red, green and blue, are used outside rooms and wards.

The Operating Theatre. Diffused light with no glare is necessary, and over the operating table strong shadowless lighting.

Theatres should have a second method of lighting available for use in emergency.

Factories and Schools. Lighting is very important, and in the modern buildings is studied and designed with great care. In classrooms bad lighting may do much harm to children's sight, and in factories may cause fatigue and accidents. Some important points are: glare is bad, either direct or reflected, as it makes the sight less sensitive; strong local patches of light are bad; dull lighting is a strain on the eyes and is also depressing; shadows should not be thrown across working tables or desks—in factories this is very dangerous. (For illustration of classroom lighting, see p. 259.)

Lighting in the Home. Where selection is possible, as in new houses, the lighting scheme should be chosen with care. The aim should be to give a pleasing effect, as well as to have really good lighting where it is most wanted. The wall colourings must be taken into account, because any of the shades in the second half of the list on page 54 will require considerably stronger lighting.

The Living Room. It is essential to have good local lighting where reading, writing, study or sewing are carried on. Floor or table adjustable standard lights should be placed in these positions, in addition to a general hanging light with a diffused or under-shade. A dining table, wherever placed, needs a good central light.

The Kitchen. Fluorescent strip lighting, because it is shadowless, is by far the most suitable since the housewife must be continually moving between the cooker, the work-table and the sink. If that is not possible good individual lights should be over each of these fixtures.

Bedrooms. Reading lamps should be sufficiently tall and so shaded that light will fall conveniently on a book. Dressing-table lights should be placed with suitable regard for their purpose.

Bathroom. Fluorescent lighting is very suitable. If lamps are used they are placed close to the ceiling, enclosed in opaque bowl shades so that steam cannot damp the flex. Filament tubular lamps are useful for placing at the sides of mirrors.

Entrance. A light should be provided outside the front door to light up steps and numbers, as well as hall lights inside.

Streets and Exteriors. *Streets.* Lighting is of great importance in prevention of road accidents. Since objects in the road show up in contrast to their background the aim of good street-lighting is to produce a uniformly bright background. The colour of objects, so useful in daytime, does not help at night. A very efficient lighting is by high-pressure arc lamps (in a vacuum tube), filled with mercury vapour for a bluish light, or sodium vapour for a yellowish light.

Illumination Tubes for Decoration and Advertising. Tubes are filled with gas, which glows when the current is switched on. Neon gives a red glow; argon, blue; mercury vapour in a brown glass tube gives green, etc.

Floodlighting is used for display and for night work, as in docks, yards, buildings under construction, etc. Beams of light are thrown out by projectors, and if the surface of the building is dirty and reflection poor, two-thirds of the lighting effect may be lost. For colour floodlighting gas-filled tubes are used, and to give a great brilliancy the luminous vapour in them can be put under high pressure (150 atmospheres).

Other Methods of Lighting.

Gas. Coal gas is a mixture of gases including hydrogen, carbon dioxide, nitrogen, methane and carbon monoxide. It is obtained from coal by distillation.

It is now used for lighting only where electricity is not available. It adds many products of combustion to the air, including carbon dioxide, water vapour and carbon monoxide (the cause of coal-gas poisoning). One burner contaminates the air with carbon dioxide to the same extent as the breathing of four people.

Incandescent burners contaminate the air less and give a better light. They consist of bunsen burners over which hang asbestos mantles which when heated become brightly luminous.

Oil Lamps.   Paraffin in the well of the lamp soaks up the wick, and gives off an inflammable vapour (hence the wick-holder must screw in tightly to avoid explosion).   The best lamps have an incandescent mantle, and an automatic extinguisher in case of overturning.   The lighting is poor, and products of combustion cause an unpleasant smell.   The products are smoke (carbon particles), carbon dioxide, water vapour, and certain volatile substances.   Pressure oil lamps with a mantle give a good light and do not smell but make a noise, which some people find disturbing.

Candles have a low lighting power.   The products of combustion are the same as those of oil, but in negligible quantities.

CHAPTER IV

WATER SUPPLY

THE water supply of a country is of vital importance. For drinking it must be a pure water supply, and to ensure this, especially in large cities, is a tremendous scientific and engineering achievement.

Contamination of Water

Pure water to a chemist means sterile distilled water, that is, steam condensed and collected in a sterile vessel.

"Pure" drinking water has in it mineral salts, dissolved from the soil through which it has passed. It is clear, sparkling, colourless, and without sediment, and above all it contains *no harmful* (*pathogenic*) *bacteria*.

The pathogenic bacteria that may contaminate water are the organisms of:

> Typhoid and paratyphoid fever.
> Dysentery.
> Cholera, in tropical countries.

These organisms are present in the excreta of patients or carriers and any leakage of sewage into the water supply is liable to start an epidemic.

Outbreaks of these waterborne diseases therefore are always due to *sewage pollution*, and this may occur from leakages in drains, cesspools or sewage tanks, from privies near shallow wells, or from insufficiently purified effluent in streams.

It follows that water supply schemes are closely concerned with drainage works.

Other organic impurities of less importance are decaying vegetation and the eggs of certain worms in tropical countries.

The only mineral that may make water harmful is lead, dissolved from pipes if the water is acid due to peaty moorland vegetation. Lead poisoning may result, but is avoided by putting lime or chalk in the reservoirs in order to make the water alkaline so that lead will not be dissolved.

The salts dissolved up from the rock layers through which the water has passed are not impurities in drinking water, but rather improve it, though they may make it hard.

The water supply of a country depends on its rainfall and on the arrangement of its layers of rock at the surface and deep underground.

Water evaporated from sea and land condenses in the higher atmosphere and falls again as rain, snow or hail on the surface soil beneath which the rock may be permeable or impermeable.

Permeable rocks, chiefly sandstone and chalk hold water well. Rain soaks into surface layers, finds its way into deep layers, where water collects in great underground lakes.

Limestone also lets water through, being full of cracks and fissures. Examples of *impermeable rocks* are clay and granite. Water cannot pass through these, but collects in the permeable layers above.

Sources from which Water Supplies are Obtained

1. Upland Surface Water Lakes.

In mountainous regions natural lakes are used to provide the water supply for cities often far distant. A dam is built across the valley to hold back the water and enlarge the lake which is then called an *impounding reservoir*. The water is piped to the towns to be supplied and is spoken of as *upland surface water*. The lake is fed by the rainfall on the surrounding mountains flowing down in streams and water channels. The water is soft, because it is surface water which has not been deep enough in the earth to dissolve mineral salts.

Its *purity* depends on supervision of the mountain sides which receive the rainfall. This land, called the *catchment area*, is the property of the Water Board concerned, so that it can be suitably controlled. Farms and houses are not allowed on it, though it may be let for cattle grazing, and usually it is fenced in except for a few well-defined paths. The purity of the water is thus assured.

This is the water that may be slightly acid if the catchment area is peaty moorland, in which case it may be treated as explained above.

Big water schemes that include impounding reservoirs are to be found in many countries. A few examples are:

Lake Vyrnwy in North Wales which is five miles long and supplies Liverpool with water; the Elan Valley Lake in Wales supplying Birmingham; enormous dams in the mountains near Bombay which form "monsoon lakes" to store the monsoon rain water to be used for water power, irrigation and water supply for Bombay. The Owen Falls Dam on the Nile raises the level of Lake Victoria by 6 feet, and provides for irrigation in the valley of the Nile at all seasons. It also provides power for a hydro-electric power station supplying Uganda with electricity.

Pipe lines and aqueducts convey these water supplies to the cities. Aqueducts built of concrete, or pipes made of cast iron or, more lately, of steel lead the water to the water works and pumping stations. Some of the big aqueducts are 8 to 12 feet in diameter and miles in length, and the water mains under the roads of cities are about 4 feet in diameter.

2. Wells.

Wherever the surface rock is permeable, *e.g.*, sandstone, chalk or limestone, the rain water trickles through, and collects as vast underground lakes on the surface of a lower layer of impermeable rock such as clay, through which it cannot pass. Wells are sunk into these underground lakes.

Shallow Wells. These are sunk through a permeable surface layer tapping the water collecting on the first impermeable layer of rock.

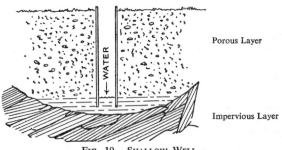

Porous Layer

Impervious Layer

Fig. 19.—Shallow Well.

They are liable to be grossly polluted from privies, middens, farm buildings, cesspools, and manure and refuse heaps. Contamination from these sources soaks down with the subsoil water and reaches the well water, or may enter through the side of the well higher up if it is not properly built. Outbreaks of typhoid fever in villages have often been traced to shallow wells.

The water is clear and pleasant to drink, even when dangerous.

Examples are found in every village in England and elsewhere.

Deep Wells. These are those that are sunk through a layer of impervious rock, tapping water collected on a deeper impervious layer. This water is practically safe from contamination, having been purified on its long journey through the earth from some distant part where the deep rock layers are tilted up to the surface and are open to rainfall. The water is pleasant to drink, clear and sparkling, and is usually very hard owing to the salts it has dissolved from the soil.

The names *shallow* and *deep* do not refer to the depth in feet of the wells, but to the layers or rock through which the boring is carried.

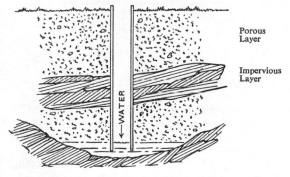

Porous Layer

Impervious Layer

WATER

FIG. 20.—DEEP WELL.

Artesian Wells (so called from Artois in France). These are very deep wells. Lengths of iron tubing, screwed on consecutively, are bored through the earth till water is reached on a deep rock layer. This layer comes to the surface on hills many miles away, and the deep water is under such pressure that it rises up without pumping.

Deep below London is a big underground lake on a clay bed. There are many privately owned wells, 400 to 600 feet deep, that tap this water. They are constructed of iron tubing driven into the ground by drilling, and are called "driven wells" or "boreholes".

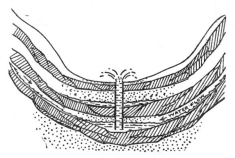

Fig. 21.—Artesian Well.

Construction of " Dug " Wells. The walls of brick set in cement should go down at least 20 feet, and if possible penetrate to the water.

A layer of concrete should surround the upper 6 feet.

A coping is formed by the brick wall rising 2 feet above ground.

A concrete platform should surround the coping, sloping away from the well.

A cover should be over the top.

A pump should be fixed (instead of chain and bucket) as soon as water is reached.

There should be no source of contamination near the well, especially on a higher slope.

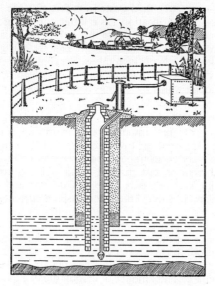

Fig. 22.—An EFFICIENTLY CONSTRUCTED "DUG WELL".

3. Rivers.

River water comes from upland surface water and from springs, both deep and surface. A *surface spring* is subsoil water from permeable rock escaping at the surface and is liable to contamination. The water of *deep* or *main springs* is pure and hard like that of deep wells. The water may find a natural outlet gushing out as a spring where the deep strata reach the surface.

River water in the upper reaches is contaminated from farms, manured fields, sewage of villages and animal pollution. After passing through towns and cities it is further contaminated by effluent from sewage works (though this must reach a specified standard of

3

purity—see p. 87), fluid waste from factories, etc. After processes of purification river water can be used for water supplies. For example, from the Thames and its tributaries London uses about 140,000,000 gallons daily—two-thirds of the total water supply.

The degree of hardness depends on the nature of the soil through which the springs that feed it have passed.

4. Rain Water.

This is of great importance in many hot countries where it is stored for town supplies and for irrigation. Storage may be in impounded reservoirs or in underground cement cisterns fed from sloping concrete collecting surfaces as is done in Gibraltar and Aden. In England it is used chiefly for washing purposes since it is very soft. If it is collected from the roof it will at first be contaminated with soot, etc.

Robert's Separator is an apparatus which automatically tips out the first water collected, and passes the rest into a tank. As rain falls through the air it takes into solution a certain amount of carbon dioxide as well as fine particles of substances present in the air.

5. Distilled Sea Water.

This is used on ships to supplement the fresh water carried. It is flat to the taste and needs aerating.

Methods of Purifying Water

The following are the methods in use, with their points of advantage and disadvantage:

1. Boiling.

This is suitable only for small quantities.

All organisms are killed after a few minutes' boiling.

Hard water is made soft.

It becomes flat to the taste because the gases in solution that made it sparkling are driven off, but it can be re-aerated by filling a bottle half full and shaking it well, or by pouring the water from a height of a few feet through a sieve or "rose" of a water-can into a receptacle.

2. Distillation.

Steam is passed through a tube in which it is cooled, so that it condenses, the water dropping into a recep-

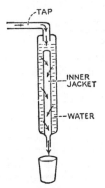

tacle. It is used on a large scale in ships, and in small quantities in dispensaries to dilute those drugs which would be affected by the presence of salts, etc., in water.

Distilled water contains no salts, since they do not pass off in steam, and is therefore flat to the taste.

It is not "sterile water" unless received in a sterile receptacle.

3. Domestic Filters.

There are two kinds: the *Berkefeld* and the *Pasteur-Chamberland*.

FIG. 23.—SECTION OF A PASTEUR-CHAMBERLAND FILTER.

The filter screws on a tap, and is shaped like a hollow candle with an inner jacket of fine porcelain. Tap water fills the outer space, and must filter through to the inner space before it can reach the outlet. The porcelain is so fine that it holds back most bacteria.

Filtration is very slow, and they are most unsatisfactory. They need to be taken to pieces, scrubbed and boiled every few days to cleanse the porcelain from organisms arrested in the outer tube, and if cracked or ill-fitting they are not only useless but dangerous.

4. Natural or Self-Purification.

In rivers, lakes and storage reservoirs water becomes purified to a large extent by the following means:

(1) Sand and other solids settle if the water moves slowly.

(2) Bacteria break up substances in solution.

(3) Protozoa (one-cell organisms) feed on organic matter and bacteria.

(4) Insect larvæ feed on protozoa and other organic matter.

(5) Fish feed on larvæ, etc.

(6) Water plants use carbon-dioxide and give out oxygen.

(7) Sunlight and air destroy bacteria.

(8) Mere storage of water causes it to become free of organisms. Typhoid bacilli in water stored in a laboratory will nearly all be dead in a week.

5. Chlorination.

Chlorine is a strong disinfectant. It is very valuable in the treatment of water supplies since it is the quickest and safest method known. It is used in all water works where river water undergoes purification in preparation for supplying towns.

After leaving the storage reservoirs and the sand filter, the water is piped to a "chlorination house", where gaseous chlorine is injected under pressure into the water in carefully measured doses which are sufficient to destroy bacteria without making the water taste of chlorine. When there is danger of serious contamination of water the dose of chlorine is increased, the taste being of minor importance.

If ammonia is added as well as chlorine, a substance *chloramine* is formed, which is an even stronger disinfectant and is tasteless.

6. Sand Filtration.

This may be carried out in two ways:

(*a*) **Filter Beds.** A filter bed is a concrete reservoir, filled in layers (see Fig. 25).

A green gelatinous film composed of algæ forms in the upper few inches of the sand. This is a growth of microscopic plant life and bacteria which removes most of the harmful bacteria in the water, while the layers below provide mechanical filtration.

The cleaning of the sand is done when the film becomes too thick (in about six to eight weeks) and

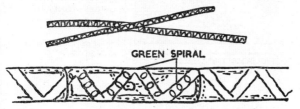

GREEN SPIRAL

FIG. 24.—DETAIL OF ALGÆ FROM A FILTER BED SHOWING MICROSCOPIC PLANT LIFE.

filtration is too slow. The water is run off, the green film removed and the sand hosed. Until a new film forms in two days or more, filtration is not efficient, so the water is filtered through this, and then through a "ripe" filter with a well developed film.

Where the water contains much debris, as for example, Thames water, a preliminary filtration through a quick sand filter may be carried out before the water is run on to the main filter bed.

(*b*) **Pressure Filters.** These are in closed concrete tanks or "boxes" instead of open reservoirs. The layers are the same, but instead of the green organic film there is a chemical film deposited on the sand. This purifies the water, which flows off through pipes at the bottom.

The process is much quicker than it is in open filter beds. Pressure filters are cleaned by forcing compressed air up through the filter layers together with clean water.

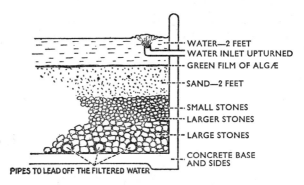

FIG. 25.—SECTION THROUGH A FILTER BED.

7. Ozone.

This is useful for purifying water (a molecule of ozone consists of three atoms of oxygen). It is produced in nature during thunderstorms by lightning passing through the air, and for commercial use for water purification, by passing oxygen through an electrical apparatus.

Swimming Baths

The water in swimming baths quickly becomes polluted with organic matter both as particles and in solution and needs constant purification; for this various types of plant are used. The water is drawn out of the bath at the deep end by a suction pump and passes through a filter screen; powerful pumps then circulate it through the purification plant. The process of purification is as follows: (1) the water undergoes chemical treatment with aluminium carbonate; (2) it is filtered through pressure filters constructed of graded layers of sand, gravel and stone, with a chemical filtering film in the upper layer of the sand; (3) the water is then warmed as it passes through a calorifier, and (4) aerated,

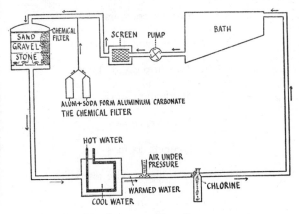

FIG. 26.—SWIMMING BATH PURIFICATION.

usually by means of air under pressure, and finally (5) it is chlorinated. It is then returned into the shallow end of the bath. The pressure filter is cleaned at intervals by upward-forcing of compressed air through the layers, thus loosening the impurities, which are then washed away into drains by an upward-forced flow of water. The bath or pool is emptied at intervals and the floor is cleaned with a suction sweeper.

DISTRIBUTION OF WATER

The course of water from *source to citizen* is—

Catchment area

|

Lake, reservoir or river

|

Water works

|

Storage reservoirs

|

Tanks for softening, if necessary

|

Filter beds or pressure filters

|

Chlorination house

|

Storage tanks

|

Pumping stations

|

Water tower or high service reservoirs

|

Cast iron water main under the road

|

Lead service pipes to house

|

Cold water pipes   Boiler for heating

The process of softening will be described later. The water is led from each stage to the next in pipes of cast iron.

Storage tanks are covered and very large.

Water Tower or Service Reservoirs. The water is pumped up to a height so that it may flow by gravity down to the town and have sufficient pressure to force it up to the upper stories of buildings.

Water mains are made of cast iron coated inside with "protective" to prevent rust, or sometimes of steel. The joints of the sections are carefully sealed, because the pipes are laid under the roads close to sewers and gas pipes.

Service pipes from the mains into houses are made of lead for easy bending or more recently of polythene. Galvanized iron or copper may be used where the water is acid.

The Supply in the House. The water in the pipes is straight from the main and is always available.

Tanks and Cisterns. These should be made of galvanized iron, slate or stoneware (never lead), covered to avoid pollution with dust, insects, mice, etc., and ventilated. They should be easy of access, and must be cleaned out at regular intervals.

The quantity allowed per head varies in different towns, 60 gallons per head is the usual average in cities.

The purposes for which it is used are:

> Drinking.
> Cooking.
> Baths (about 20 gallons each).
> Washing (personal).
> Washing dishes and cleaning.
> Water closet (3 gallons each time the cistern is
>   emptied).
> Watering gardens.
> Laundry.
> Car washing.

Also each citizen's share of street cleaning and flushing sewers, public baths and swimming baths, fire extinguishing, trades and manufactures and agriculture.

Also a certain amount of waste.

Waste. It should be remembered that water is expensive and water rates are often high. This is not surprising considering the expense of upkeep of such

3*

vast engineering schemes. Hospitals pay large sums each year for water, and therefore waste should be avoided. Nurses should see that any leaking taps or perished washers are reported and repaired, and that taps are turned off and not left running.

Meters are installed to record the amount of water used.

HARDNESS OF WATER

Water is *hard* when it contains excess salts of calcium or magnesium. Bicarbonate of calcium (lime) and magnesium can be removed from water by boiling; this is sometimes called *temporary hardness*. Sulphates of calcium and magnesium can also be removed, but not by boiling; this was formerly spoken of as *permanent hardness*, but the term is not correct.

The water has dissolved these salts from the rocks through which it has passed.

Bicarbonate of lime is the salt that makes water hard in regions where the rock is chalk, *e.g.* the North and South Downs. Chalk (carbonate of lime) is not soluble in water, but if more carbon is combined with it, *bicarbonate of lime* is formed, which is readily soluble in water. This happens when rain water soaks and trickles through chalk soil. The carbon dioxide in the rain water provides the extra carbon which unites with the chalk to make bicarbonate of lime and the water of the springs and wells will be hard.

The following methods will remove this salt and make the water soft:

1. Boiling. The extra carbon dioxide will be driven off, leaving insoluble carbonate of lime, which is precipitated in kettles, pipes and boilers, forming a hard crust known as "fur" or "scale".

2. Adding Lime. This will have the same result. The fresh lime takes some of the carbon from the bicarbonate of lime so that chalk is produced in large amounts and is precipitated.

Further methods of softening that remove all hardening salts are:

3. Adding Soda. Chemical reactions take place and the hardening salts are precipitated.

4. The Permutit Process. A cylinder (small for the home, large for an institution), containing a layer of mineral substance known as zeolites, is attached to the cold water supply. As the water runs through, by a chemical process the zeolite removes all the hardening salts. When the zeolite has become saturated with lime and other salts it is flushed through with a strong solution of brine to clean it, followed by water to rinse it, and then it is ready for use again.

5. Using an Excessive Amount of Soap. When soap is used with hard water it will not lather, but the fatty acids in it combine with lime in the water and make curds. Eventually if enough soap were used, a lather could be produced.

Disadvantages of Hard Water

1. It is wasteful with soap.
2. It is bad for the skin.
3. The curds may block up sink pipes.
4. It "furs" kettles and boilers and steam pipes with three results:

> (a) water takes much longer to heat, so there is waste of coal and gas.
>
> (b) in boilers so much overheating may cause the boiler plates to burst. Boilers in hospitals, factories, public buildings and ships are inspected regularly; the plates should have a thin layer of "scale" inside.
>
> (c) steam pipes become gradually blocked up with "fur" or "scale".

5. It is bad for cooking vegetables and making tea.
6. A ring of sticky scum is left round the bath, to be scoured off.

CHAPTER V

SANITATION
DRAINAGE AND REFUSE DISPOSAL

THE disposal of sewage is a problem of extreme interest and it has been developed, by long scientific research through successive stages, to its present high degree of efficiency whereby the sewage of great cities is rendered harmless and finally disposed of without any unpleasant smells and, what is far more important, without polluting the water supplies. Ultimately a large volume of the sewage of big towns is discharged into rivers, and if it were not for the processes of purification there would be outbreaks of the waterborne diseases—*typhoid fever*, *dysentery* and, in some countries, *cholera*.

There are five types of refuse:

1. Excreta.
2. Waste water from sinks, baths, etc.
3. Surface water—rain and street washings.
4. Trade waste from factories.
5. House refuse (including hospital refuse).

Drainage and Sewage Disposal are concerned with the first four.

In towns which have a sufficient water supply, all types of waste are conveyed to the sewage disposal works by the *water carriage system.*

In country places, many dwellings still use the *conservancy system.*

The Water-carriage System

The first stage is the carrying of excreta, waste water and rain water to the sewer by means of pipes and drains. Here it is joined by storm water (on occasion), waste from gas and electrical works, dairies, etc. and, in industrial towns, many types of factory waste.

The system consists of:

A. **Collecting Places.** Lavatory pans, baths, sinks and sluices, washing basins.

B. **Overground Pipes.** Soil pipe, waste-water pipe, rain-water pipe, anti-siphonage pipe.

C. **Underground Drains.** House drain, sewer.

D. **Sewage Disposal Works.**

E. **Outfall.**

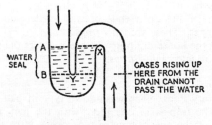

FIG. 27.—SECTION OF A TRAP.

In various positions in these pipes and drains traps are placed.

A **trap** is a device to prevent gas from decomposing sewage passing back up from the drain into the house. The commonest type is constructed by simply bending a pipe, so that in the bend water always remains, separating the air below it from that above. Thus gases cannot pass back from the sewer or drain into the house. The shape of the bend may be ⌣ or

Water remains in the trap up to the level of bend X. Should the water level fall below bend Y, gas could pass, and the trap is then said to be "*unsealed*". The water between A and B is therefore called the *water-seal*. It should be not less than 2 inches deep.

Traps may be unsealed by:

1. Evaporation in the very hot weather in an empty house where the pipes are not flushed.

2. Siphonage, or sucking out of the water from the trap of a lavatory pan by a rush of water down the soil pipe from a floor above. (This is prevented by an anti-siphonage pipe.)

Traps are placed in the following positions:

1. Under every lavatory pan, bath, sink, sluice and washing basin.

2. Under the open ends of waste-water and rain-water pipes. These are *gully traps*.

3. In the house drain just before it enters the sewer. These are *intercepting traps*.

A. Collecting Places

Lavatory Pans. The wash-down type of pan is the best. The trap is in one piece with the pan, and a branch of the anti-siphonage pipe opens into the top of the trap. The pipe passes through the wall and joins

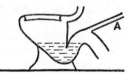

FIG. 28.—WASH-DOWN PAN WITH TRAP IN ONE PIECE.
A—branch to anti-siphonage pipe.

the soil pipe with a carefully sealed joint. The pan has a water rim to distribute the water over the whole surface. The flush should be 3 gallons or, at least, 2 gallons. The material is glazed stoneware, and the pedestal is not enclosed. The lavatory must have an outside wall against which the pedestal is placed. There must be a window, which will open, in area not less than 2 square feet, and the walls and floor should be washable.

Baths and Wash-basins. These are made of porcelain enamel and many new types are of pressed steel porcelain-enamelled in pastel shades. Baths are either raised on feet with space around for cleaning or built in completely.

The waste pipe is trapped, and leads into the wastewater pipe. There must be an overflow pipe.

The bathroom should have an outside wall, a window, and washable walls and floor.

Sinks. Most of the new models are made of stainless steel or of pressed steel porcelain-enamelled in pastel shades. They are usually combined to form a unit with draining boards and cabinet cupboards, and some with a refrigerator as well. They are easy to keep clean, and look very attractive. Older types are of glazed stoneware.

The trap in the pipe under the sink has a *cleaning screw* at the lowest bend which can be removed for cleaning the trap if it gets blocked. The pipe leads into the waste-water pipe, and there must be an overflow pipe.

B. Overground Pipes

On the side or back walls of a building four varieties of pipes may be observed:

1. Large pipes that run straight into the ground and go high above the roof gutter, with wire caged tops. Branches joining the main pipe slope downwards.

These are **soil pipes** from the water-closets.

2. Pipes with wire caged tops high above the roof gutter but open at the lower end over gully traps in the ground. Branch pipes slope downwards.

These are **waste-water pipes** from *baths, sinks, washing basins,* etc.

Several pipes may sometimes be arranged to come together on the wall and empty into a single pipe running down thus:

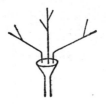

Fig. 29.—Branch Pipes into a Single Pipe.

3. Pipes coming from the roof gutter opening at the lower end over gully traps, and having no branches.

These are **rain-water pipes.**

Actually pipes 2 and 3 often go into the ground, appearing like soil pipes, but just below ground level they turn and open under the iron grating above the gully trap.

4. Much smaller pipes near soil pipes which do not go down to the ground. The upper end may (*a*) go above the roof with a cage, or (*b*) open into the soil pipe high up.

The lower end may (*a*) be a closed end on the wall, or (*b*) open into the soil pipe below the lowest lavatory.

Branches which come from the traps of lavatory pans enter at an upward slope.

These are **anti-siphonage pipes.**

The Anti-siphonage Pipe. This is designed to prevent the unsealing of traps. Lavatories on several floors are often one above the other and their branch pipes go into the same soil pipe. When one of the upper pans is flushed, the 3 gallons of water rushing down the soil pipe, past the openings of lower branches, causes a suction action, due to the vacuum created behind the falling water. The suction might draw the water out of the traps of the lower lavatory pans, leaving them unsealed, but this is prevented by the anti-siphonage pipe. It has branches containing *air* connected to the top of each of these traps, so that any suction in the soil

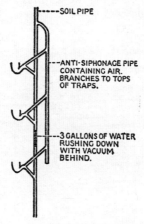

FIG. 30.—ANTI-SIPHONAGE PIPE.

pipe draws air from the latter, instead of water from the trap.

The One-Pipe System.   This is a modern method in which there is only one pipe for excreta and waste water. All collecting places—lavatory pans, baths, sinks, etc.—must be trapped with special 3-inch deep seal traps, and the lower end of the pipe goes straight into the ground, to pass into the house drain in an inspection chamber. This system is becoming increasingly popular.

Details of Pipes 1, 2 and 3

1. Soil Pipe.	2. Waste-Water Pipe.	3. Rain-Water Pipe.
Contains only excreta. Must be on the outside of the wall. Made of cast iron or lead. Size : 3 to 6 inches diameter (not less). Lengths of pipe are fixed together with spigot and socket joints. Joints of iron pipes are sealed with molten lead to prevent escape of gases. Branches are from lavatory pans and sluices only and enter at a downward slope, never at right angles. Upper end is above the roof gutter but not near windows or roof gardens. It is caged to prevent blockage with birds' nests, etc. The pipe is straight, or if a bend is necessary it is an "easy" bend (not sharp). Lower end goes straight into the ground and there turns and slopes towards the the sewer, changing its name to "house drain". There is frequently an anti-siphonage pipe connected with it.	Contains waste water. Branches enter it from baths, sinks, lavatory basins, etc. Diameter, 2 to 4 inches. Lower end opens over a gully trap, either above or under the grating. Leads into the house drain at an inspection chamber.	Comes from the roof gutter. Has no branches and no anti-siphonage pipe. Opens over a trapped gully.

C. Underground Pipes

Continuing at a slope, a few feet underground, run (a) the soil pipe, having changed its name to *house drain*, (b) one or more pipes from any nearby gully traps (containing waste and rain water). These pipes converge, and meet in an *inspection chamber*.

1. The Inspection Chamber.—This has an iron cover flush with the ground. When this is raised a cement-lined manhole is seen, with the openings of the above pipes on one or two sides. The pipes pass across the floor as open "half channels" of glazed earthenware, all leading into a single drain pipe, on the opposite side, which is the house drain continued. The excreta and waste water are washed across to this pipe through the half channels, the flow of water being sufficient to keep them clean, although they are periodically inspected and disinfected. The purpose of the inspection chamber is to make possible inspection of pipes where several converge.

2. The House Drain starts where the soil pipe, after entering the ground, changes its direction and slopes towards the sewer. It passes through an inspection chamber as a half channel and is here joined by the water pipes (as explained above). It then continues at a slope, containing all excreta and waste water. It is made in sections, either of glazed stoneware jointed with cement, or iron jointed with lead, and is laid in cement. Just before entering the sewer it is trapped with an *intercepting trap*, and at this point there is an *intercepting chamber*.

3. The Intercepting Trap and Chamber. Near the sewer is a deep cement-lined manhole with an airtight but removable cover and a cement base. Across the bottom passes the house drain, which is trapped at this point to prevent sewer air passing up into the drain. This intercepting trap has an opening, the "raking arm" closed with a screw stopper through which the section of drain to the sewer may be cleaned.

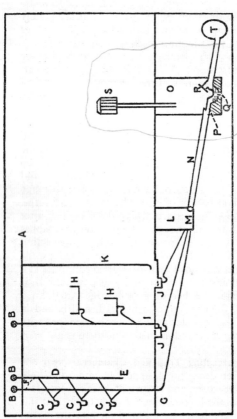

FIG. 31.—OUTLINE OF WATER-CARRIAGE SYSTEM OF DRAINAGE.

A, Roof line; B, caged openings of pipes; C, C, C, lavatory pans with traps; D, anti-siphonage pipe with E closed end and F alternative opening; G, soil pipe entering ground—*no* trap; H, H, bath and sink, both trapped; I, waste-water pipe opening into trapped gully; J, J, gully traps; K, rain-water pipe; L, inspection chamber with movable cover; M, pipes pass across as half channels; N, house drain; O, intercepting chamber with air-tight stone cover; P, drain as a half channel laid in cement; Q, intercepting trap showing water seal; R, raking arm with screw cap; S, ventilator with mica flap against wall; T, sewer.

From the near side of the trap a ventilating shaft leads up to the open air, to ventilate the house drain. It is usually fixed against a nearby wall, and is often fitted with an Arnott's ventilator.

4. The Sewer. This usually runs under the road, and leads out of the town to the sewage disposal works. House drains from all the houses open into it, and in big towns small sewers empty into deep main sewers. Small sewers are stoneware or concrete pipes jointed with cement or iron jointed with lead. Large ones are of concrete or brickwork set in cement and are round or egg-shaped. They are always ventilated. Sewer air in properly ventilated sewers is not dangerous and does not spread disease. Bacteria such as typhoid bacilli, if present, are in the fluid sewage, and not in the air. Leaking sewers or drains would be highly dangerous as water pipes run near them under the road, and the water might be infected through leaking joints. This has, in fact, happened at times, and outbreaks of typhoid fever have occurred in this way.

D. Sewage Disposal

Sewers carry to the sewage disposal works:

> Excreta and waste water from buildings.
> Surface water (rain and street washings).
> Waste from factories and municipal works.

Sometimes a large main sewer carries it all, with perhaps the addition of "overflows" to carry off storm water, or there may be a separate sewer for the surface water in districts where there are many big tarred or concrete roads.

Liquid waste from factories must be accepted (by an Act passed in 1937) for disposal in the public sewers, but, if it is not suitable, the Sanitary Authority may order it first to be diluted or treated.

E. Outfalls

Eventually the sewerage reaches the sea, a river or a large lake, but only after it has been sufficiently purified to prevent pollution of the water.

The Sea. Discharge of crude sewage into the sea is getting less common. The amount of treatment it undergoes depends on the direction of sea currents and the position of bathing beaches. At least screening and sedimentation are usually carried out.

Big Lakes. These may receive sewage, but complete treatment is necessary for all lakeside towns.

Rivers. Except in the case of very small towns on very large rivers, a full treatment is usually required.

Sewage Treatment

A full treatment consists of:

A. Preliminary Treatment

The crude sewage carried to the works by the main sewer is a fluid consisting of *water* containing *domestic sewage* (*i.e.* excreta and other waste from houses); *sand* and *road grit* carried by the rainfall through gutters and drains; *paper*, *rags*, *etc.* that have been washed into the sewer; and *trade waste* from factories, dairies, gasworks and other industries.

This crude sewage flows first through an **iron grid** or **screen** where coarse rubbish such as rags, sticks, paper etc. are caught and held. Mechanical rakes clean the screen and the waste is used for compost, or burned. The sewage then flows into narrow open channels where it moves very slowly so that grit may settle; these are the **grit channels** or **detritus tanks**. The settled grit in modern works is washed free of organic matter and dumped on land, or it may be buried or burned.

From the grit channels the sewage flows along **feed channels** into **sedimentation tanks** with sloping floors where in a few hours much of the solid material settles to the bottom. This sediment is called **sludge,** and the liquid is **effluent.** There may be a second set of these tanks where yet more sludge settles. The effluent flows on, and it is this liquid which, after further purification, is allowed to go into the river. The sludge is pumped out of the tanks and disposed of separately.

To repeat: Preliminary treatment of crude sewage consists of: (1) **Screening.** (2) Passing through **grit channels.** (3) Remaining for some hours in **sedimentation tanks,** where it separates into effluent and sludge. Since the effluent is to be discharged into a river, its further purification is very important.

B. Purification

Effluent still contains a large amount of organic matter, which must be broken down into harmless salts—nitrates, nitrites, etc.—before it can be discharged into a stream. This work is done by bacteria and they need an ample supply of oxygen, so for this final stage the sewage must be brought into contact with millions of bacteria and plentifully supplied with air.

There are two methods of doing this: 1. The percolating filter method. 2. The activated sludge method. In both cases the final effluent discharging into the river must be clear and must reach the required standard of purity. Samples are tested at intervals to ensure this.

The Percolating Filter Method. The effluent from the sedimentation tank is piped to a **biological filter** which is open and circular, built of concrete, about 6 feet deep, and filled with coke, small clinker or stones, thus containing a plentiful supply of air.

A gelatinous film covers every stone or clinker, and in this millions of bacteria multiply, being well supplied with oxygen. Over the surface a steel pipe rotates, from which the effluent is sprinkled on to the clinker, and as it trickles through, the bacteria and protozoa in the film break down the impurities and oxidise them. The process is helped by the larvæ of "filter flies" and midges that feed on the sewage. These flies do not carry disease organisms, and so are harmless.

Some of the film of bacterial and plant life is washed off into the effluent, forming a dark brown muddy deposit called humus. This must not pass into the river, so the outflow pipe from the bottom of the filter leads to a **humus tank** where the flow is slowed down for the humus to settle, after which the cleared effluent is discharged into the river.

The Activated Sludge Method. In this newer method there is no filter but, instead, the effluent from the sedimentation tank is passed into **aeration tanks** where bacteria act on it, breaking down organic solids in the same way as in the film that covers the filter stones. Oxygen is provided by pumping air up through perforated plates in the floor of the tank, and in some works by large paddles that stir up the sewage and mix it with air.

In about six hours the process of purification is complete and the sewage passes to a **settlement tank** where the sludge quickly settles to the bottom, and the effluent now sufficiently pure, is run off over a weir into the river. This sludge, full of active bacteria, is called activated sludge, and some of it is pumped back to the aeration tanks to mix with the fresh incoming sewage, so providing the bacterial culture required.

The remaining sludge, together with that from the earlier sedimentation tanks, is pumped off and removed for final disposal.

Sludge Disposal. In both methods, after the now harmless effluent has been discharged into the river, there remain large quantities of sludge for final disposal. The sludge is over 90 per cent. water so first it must be dried. The simplest way of doing this is by spreading it on drying beds in the open air, but this requires a

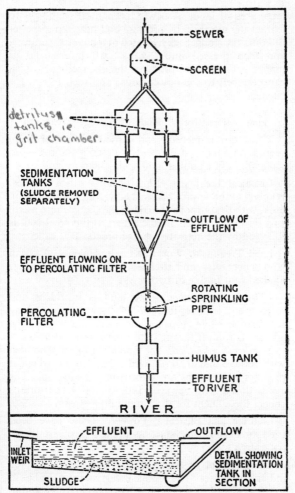

FIG. 32.—DIAGRAM OF A SMALL SEWAGE DISPOSAL WORKS WITH BIOLOGICAL FILTER.

large area of land. A newer mechanical method is to extract the moisture by pressure and heat. In a matter of hours the sludge is dehydrated at a high temperature, and then pressed into "cakes" which are sold as manure. The process produces the gas, methane, which can be piped to the power house and used to run gas engines.

Some Alternative Methods of Sewage Treatment

These are numerous and varied. Most of them require preliminary treatment as described above—*i.e.*, screening, grit chamber, and sedimentation tank.

Chemical Treatment. Lime or some other chemical is added to the sewage before it enters the sedimentation tank, with the purpose of making the sludge more useful as a fertilizer and the fluid cleaner. If this treatment is followed by the activated sludge process it is called:

Land Treatment. For this method plenty of cheap land is necessary, and after sedimentation the sewage is applied to it in one of two ways:

1. *Irrigation Method.* The land is in ridges and furrows and is under-drained. The sewage is run along the furrows while crops are grown on the ridges. The effluent is run off through the drains into a stream.

2. *Filtration Method.* The land is periodically flooded with sewage and then allowed a rest during which it recovers while crops are grown on it. After this it is again dosed with sewage, and so on. Under-drains collect the effluent for discharge into a stream.

Chlorine and Bleaching Powder. These have been tried for sterilizing sewage, but are too expensive to use on a large scale.

The Cesspool System. This is frequently used for individual houses. The sewage is carried from the house to the cesspool or septic tank by pipes, an intercepting trap being placed just before discharge into the cesspool, in order to prevent gases passing up the drain.

The cesspool should be watertight, and is usually constructed of brickwork set in cement and surrounded by puddled clay. As the sewage collects in it a leathery scum forms on the top of the fluid, and underneath this anaerobic bacteria are digesting it. When the cesspool fills up it has to be emptied. This is done by suction into mobile sewage tanks which take it to sewage works for disposal, or it may be run on to land where aerobic bacteria convert it into harmless products. The cesspool should be covered over and ventilated through a pipe opening at some height, or at some distance from the nearest dwelling.

Contamination of Water by Sewage

Excreta is liable at any time to contain the bacilli of typhoid or dysentery, and sewage may in the following ways reach the underground water which percolates into shallow wells and surface springs:

    (a) Leakage from sewers.

    (b) Cracks in tanks at sewage works.

    (c) Faulty connections.

    (d) Insufficiently purified effluent entering a stream.

    (e) Drainage from sludge-drying beds, soaking through fissures in the soil. This is a great problem, and it has been necessary in some cases to provide a bed of clay under the whole sludge-drying bed to ensure keeping the underground water supply pure.

If an outbreak of typhoid fever is traced to water *there must be sewage contamination at some point*. Samples of water from suspect wells or streams will be sent for laboratory examination and search be made to discover the source of infection.

The Conservancy System

This method is used where there is no water-carriage system with flushing tanks for water closets and sewer or cesspool to receive the sewage.

The closet in the conservancy system is called a **privy.** Privies must be at least 40 feet from any well or stream, and 6 feet from the house. There must be a window, or good ventilator, and the floor must be of cement sloping down from the receptacle to the door. Types of receptacles are:

1. Fixed Receptacles. The excreta falls into a cemented water-tight cavity under a wooden seat. It must not be bigger than 8 cubic feet; waste water must not be put in it; ashes should be thrown on the excreta; it must be emptied frequently.

2. Pails. These stand under the seat, and receive the excreta, which should be covered with ashes. The pails are changed for clean ones each week or oftener.

3. Earth Closets. In these earth is applied instead of ashes, so that the bacteria in the soil may decompose the fæcal matter. The receptacle is changed or cleaned out as above.

4. Privy Middens. In these excreta falls into a hole in the ground. The hole extends under the wall of the privy, forming an ashpit or midden on the other side of the privy wall. Excreta and refuse are thus mixed, and the fluid from it soaks through the soil and into the water of any nearby well, which will be grossly contaminated. This type of privy is highly dangerous.

Disposal of the Contents of Receptacles. The usual method is to dig it into the soil in specially dug trenches or in gardens at a distance from the house and well.

Disposal of Waste Water. The pipes from baths and sinks should lead into small drainpipes which end underground in a field or garden, about a foot down, so that the water irrigates the soil.

Chemical System

A recent development is the treatment of sewage in the container by chemicals which render it odourless and harmless. This makes possible the sanitation of aircraft where space is small and food stores, closets and travel compartments must be near together. Chemical closets are also useful for indoor and outdoor sanitation where there is no main drainage. The container in which the chemical acts on the excreta may be a movable pail under the seat and pan, or a fixed tank with an emptying valve. When fitted in a house, the tank may be drained into a cesspool, and the treated sewage, being odourless and harmless, may be used as manure.

REFUSE COLLECTION AND DISPOSAL

A large proportion of the waste matter collected from houses as "refuse" has a considerable value, and if salvaged can be converted into raw material to save imports. This is a matter of great importance in the national economy.

Household Bins. These are galvanized iron cylinders raised on rims from the ground. They must have close-fitting lids to keep out flies and cats. They should not be placed near kitchen, larder or nursery windows. The contents should be as dry as possible to avoid decomposition of organic matter. Household bins should be emptied once or twice a week by the town refuse collectors, and ward bins are emptied daily. They should be cleaned regularly, but disinfectants must not be used in bins for food refuse sold for pigs.

Types of Refuse. Waste materials that have value should, if possible, be kept separate, to assist the work of sorting. Local Authorities dispose of the salvaged waste to factories, sending monthly returns of quantities to the Ministry of Supply.

The chief wastes of value are:

Paper to save imported wood pulp. Bones (other than fish bones) for glue and fertilizers. Fat and grease of all kinds. Food waste of other kinds for pig feeding (not orange peel or egg shells). Fish waste for fertilizers. Iron, steel and tin articles. Rags. Bottles. Cinders should be used up in the house.

Collection. Scavenging motors or refuse carts are closed in when moving so that no dust or papers can be blown out.

Disposal. There are three methods:

(a) Separation (sorting) and incineration.

(b) Incineration only.

(c) Controlled tipping.

In England the cost of collecting and disposing of house refuse is considerable.

Incineration. The refuse is consumed at great heat, only clinker remaining. Small types of incinerators are made for houses and small hospitals, and these are excellent for organic refuse that is not usable. In hospitals there is one type of refuse, septic matter, which is collected in separate bins and must be burned in an incinerator or furnace *on the premises.*

The Garchey system of collection and incineration has been found useful in high blocks of flats. All household refuse is placed in a receptacle under the sink which connects with a system of vertical shafts leading to underground chambers and thence to the incinerator. The refuse is washed down the shaft and drawn by vacuum pumps to the incinerator, being partially dried in a centrifuge on the way. In England this system has been tried in Leeds.

Tips. With new and better methods, this has become a very popular way of disposing of dry refuse. These

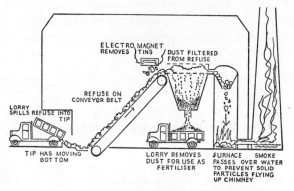

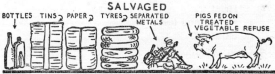

FIG. 33—REFUSE DESTRUCTION.

new methods include the so-called "Controlled System" of dumping or tipping on land. Suggested precautions issued by the Ministry of Health include:

1. Layers of refuse should not be more than 6 feet deep, and should be covered with 9 inches of earth. Not more than 100 square yards should be left uncovered at any time.

2. Screens should be put up to prevent paper, etc., being blown about by the wind.

3. No refuse may be deposited in water.

4. If the refuse contains much organic matter it should be covered by 2 feet of earth.

5. Tins, etc., should not be near the surface.

6. Each layer should be allowed to settle before the next is added.

CHAPTER VI

HYGIENE OF THE INDIVIDUAL

Personal hygiene is concerned with cleanliness and care of the body, regulation of daily life to maintain physical fitness, and habits and mental outlook.

It may be discussed under the following headings:

1. *Care and Cleanliness:*
   Skin.
   Hands and feet.
   Head.
   Mouth and teeth.
   Parasites.

2. *Physical Fitness:*
   Breathing.
   Bowels and diet.
   Clothing.   (See Chapter VIII.)
   Exercise.
   Sleep and recreation.
   Fresh air and sunlight.

3. *Habits and Mental Outlook.*

1. Care and Cleanliness

The Skin.   This is an extensive and important organ containing many nerve endings, glands and blood-vessels. Healthy skin should be firm, supple and elastic.

Its functions of—

(*a*) protection from entry of micro-organisms;
(*b*) heat regulation⎱ by its sweat glands and blood-
(*c*) excretion   ⎰   vessels; and
(*d*) formation of vitamin D by ultra-violet rays on sebum

all depend for their efficiency on its cleanliness, good blood supply and general healthy tone.

Cleanliness. Dirt on skin consists of dried sebum solids left from evaporated sweat, "dust", bacteria, and epithelial scales from its surface. All these clog the pores of the secreting glands. Washing with soap removes dirt because the alkali forms an emulsion with the oily sebum, and the dirt is washed off with it by the water.

Warm baths (temperature 100° F.) are cleansing (from secretions and dirt), refreshing, and have a sedative action due to a soothing effect on the nerve endings. They may be taken at any time.

Hot baths should be taken at night, just before going to bed, and at least an hour after a meal. The effect is to dilate all the skin blood vessels, drawing blood away from deep organs and from the brain. Depletion of the deep organs hinders digestion, and reduction of the blood supply of the brain induces sleep. They also refresh tired muscles by quickening the circulation and thus washing away fatigue products. After a very hot bath much sweat will be evaporated from the skin in order to regulate the temperature of the body.

All parts where two skin surfaces touch need specially careful attention, and after washing and drying a good powder should be used.

Dried sebum collected in the ducts of the sebaceous glands is the cause of *blackheads* or *comedones*, and these may become inflamed, producing the condition known as *acne*.

Abrasions of the skin, if they become infected, may lead to the condition of *impetigo*, which is spread by constant scratching and reinfection, as in the case of a child with pediculi capitis or scabies.

Blood Supply and Tone. The important work of regulating the temperature of the body depends on the response of blood vessels and sweat glands to nerve messages. The blood supply to the skin therefore has

4

the two functions of nourishing it and providing for heat loss both by radiation and sweat production.

A good blood supply is encouraged by exercise, friction, massage for the sick, and cold baths for the healthy.

Cold baths should be taken in the morning. After the preliminary contraction of skin blood vessels in response to the cold water, the circulation should quicken and the skin then shares in the glowing stimulation. The tonic effect is increased, if taken in the sea, by fresh air and salt.

Sunlight and fresh air have a very vital effect on the skin, as described in the next section. A layer of air must always surround the skin to absorb sweat, and the stimulating effect of moving air on the skin is very valuable.

The Hands. These should be kept free from cracks and roughness due to cold wind or constant use of antiseptic solutions. Suitable applications may be necessary. Hands should be kept clean and nails trimmed in a curve. Nurses should never have pointed or painted nails. They should avoid cutting the protective cuticle in such a way as to cause ragged ends, and especially punctures through which bacteria can gain entrance. *Paronychia* (whitlow) may be caused in this way.

Roughness is often caused by insufficient drying in cold weather, and by frequent "scrubbing up". The epidermis becomes dry and cracked, and in the cracks the dermis is exposed with its nerve endings, so that the hands are sore and inflamed. Glycerine (diluted) on account of its action of drawing fluid to it, or some skin cream which will prevent evaporation, should be used, until the cracks heal.

The Feet. These must be kept scrupulously clean by a daily bath (or, if that is impossible, daily washing) and careful drying between the toes.

Toe-nails should be cut horizontally because, if curved, the skin around will be pressed over the nail, and the pressure of the nail on this enfolding skin will cause the symptoms usually attributed to "ingrowing toe-nail". The feet contain many sweat glands, and excessive sweating, or *hyperidrosis*, necessitates frequent washing and change of socks or stockings. *Bromidrosis* is excessive sweating with offensive odour and soreness of the feet. The odour is due to decomposition of sweat. For this condition the feet should be washed several times a day in boric acid solution, dried, dabbed, with methylated spirit, and powdered with starch and boric powder. Stockings and shoes must be changed each time, used stockings washed, and shoes aired. Cork soles are good, and should be washed with a spirit lotion.

Corns. These are caused by pressure of badly fitting shoes. The epidermis thickens and becomes horny and grows inwards to a point. If they occur between the toes, they are kept moist and are "soft corns".

Callosities. These are large areas of thickening due to pressure and friction on the under surface of the foot.

Bunions. These are formed as a result of pointed shoes. The great toe becomes bent in, producing an angle at the junction of the metatarsophalangeal joint. The head of the metatarsal is thus a projecting point on the inner border of the foot and is exposed to pressure. A callosity forms on this point of pressure and the bursa underneath becomes chronically inflamed.

Hypertrophied Nails. These are hard, horny, thickened and of a yellowish or blackish colour. They should be treated, as soon as the condition starts, by soaking in a solution of soda bicarbonate, and careful filing.

These conditions may be avoided by wearing suitable shoes.

Shoes. These should fit the feet, and should not cramp the toes. The heels should not be so high as to throw the weight forward, and they should have a base wide enough for walking with comfort. Children's shoes especially should be well made, with a straight line on the inner side.

The Arch of the Foot. The inner bony arch should be $1\frac{1}{2}$ inches from the ground. *Dropped arch* is very painful and is caused by want of tone in the leg muscles with stretching of the supporting tendons and ligaments under the arch. The chief remedies are massage of the leg muscles; a built-up sole, raised $\frac{1}{4}$ to $\frac{1}{2}$ inch on the inner side; arch supports.

The Head. Proper care of the scalp includes daily firm brushing, using a brush with sufficiently stiff bristles set wide apart, and shampooing at frequent intervals. The scalp needs a good blood supply, and massaging for a few minutes daily is of great benefit. Fresh air is stimulating to it, and to go without a hat (except in great heat) is good.

A dry scalp, *seborrhœa sicca*, is a condition of "dandruff"—that is, epithelial scales are shed in excess. Oily or soft-soap shampoos should be used. An oily scalp, *seborrhœa oleosa*, is a condition of over-active sebaceous glands. Shampoos should be drying, so will contain spirit.

Pediculi are discussed in Chapter X.

The Mouth. In the mouth there are many varieties of bacteria always present and, as a rule, a healthy mouth is capable of dealing with these. Under conditions of sepsis, however, such as carious teeth, septic tonsils, unhealthy mucous membrane or infected sinuses, the streams of bacteria constantly pouring into the mouth find there ideal conditions for growth, helped by remains of food. The tongue becomes coated, and sordes (a collection of mucus, epithelial cells, food remains and bacteria) collect round teeth and lips.

Such a mouth may give rise to parotitis, otitis media, infected sinuses, pyorrhœa, digestive troubles, infection of the respiratory passages, and, via the general circulation, rheumatic conditions and remote septic foci.

The mouth should be well rinsed with some pleasant mouth-wash such as glycerine of thymol, and a little of it used for gargling in the morning and at night after the last meal or drink.

The Teeth. At the end of the second month of fœtal life, the earliest developmental process of tooth formation is starting. Therefore care of the child's teeth actually starts with the antenatal diet of the mother.

(a) Antenatal Diet. This must contain plenty of lime, phosphorus, and vitamins A and D. Lime and phosphorus are present in milk, eggs, vegetables and fruit, and vitamins A and D in milk and butter. The diet should contain these foods daily until the baby is weaned.

(b) After birth baby should be breast fed. If artificial feeding is necessary, cod-liver oil, or one of the vitamin D products, and orange juice should be given daily. Teeth and jaws will then be strong and well developed.

(c) When teething starts, rusks should be given to chew to increase the blood supply to the jaws and assist teething. Twenty milk teeth will then be cut between the age of six months and two years.

(d) Brushing the teeth should be started as soon as they are cut. A small brush with bristles not too hard should be used, and a non-gritty tooth paste. The child should be taught to do it himself, brushing front, back and crowns of the teeth, away from the gums.

(e) Permanent teeth (thirty-two) are cut from the seventh year onwards, and from this time there should be regular dental supervision.

(f) It is important that teeth should be in an alkaline

medium, and this is provided by saliva. If sugar is allowed to remain in the mouth it ferments and acid is produced. Children therefore should not be given sweets at night after the teeth are cleaned, unless they have a drink afterwards.

(*g*) The process of dental caries is: First a yellow film forms on the teeth; this becomes thicker and is called "tartar"; remains of food collect between the teeth and bacteria cause it to ferment, producing acid which eats through the enamel; bacteria now penetrate into the more organic dentine, where sepsis advances quickly and reaches the dental pulp containing the nerves; an abscess is then formed at the root of the tooth; pyorrhœa results, and from this septic focus bacteria are carried round in the blood stream, often producing remote infections.

Parasites. These are discussed in Chapter X.

2. Physical Fitness

Breathing. This provides the only means of oxygen intake and carbon dioxide excretion. It is also one of the means by which water is excreted, since expired air is always saturated.

At each inspiration the thorax enlarges, because the following movements take place simultaneously:

> The ribs are raised up and out.
> The diaphragm descends, pressing on the abdominal viscera.
> The wall of the abdomen is forced outwards.

About 500 c.c. of air is sucked into the lungs in this way, to mix with the 2,500 c.c. already there, and re-oxygenate it, an equal quantity being expelled on expiration. If tight clothing restricts the movement of the diaphragm, insufficient ventilation of the lungs results.

Deep breathing, either in special breathing exercises, or in any other form of exercise, sucks in about 2,000 c.c. of fresh air with a corresponding output, at each respiration. Such increased ventilation of the lungs is of great benefit in body metabolism.

The nose is intended for the air inlet, and *mouth breathing is bad*. The cause should be sought and treated; it is often found to be adenoids.

Bowels and Diet. The residue of a day's food (about 6-8 oz. of fæces) should be expelled daily; otherwise it remains in the pelvic colon, which dilates as the next day's waste is added to it. Water is absorbed from this mass, and bacteria cause it to ferment, producing gases and various poisonous substances which are absorbed into the blood stream, causing headache, apathy, dirty tongue and other symptoms of ill health.

Apart from disease, the chief causes of constipation are:

1. *Wrong Diet.* That is, not enough fruit, vegetables, brown bread or oatmeal. The cellulose in these foods stimulates peristalsis, and probably vitamin B is also essential.

2. *Too Little Fluid Intake.* Several glasses of water or fruit drink each day are very helpful.

3. *Insufficient Exercise.* The muscle walls of the intestine share in the general loss of tone produced in all the body muscles by want of exercise. Peristalsis slows down, and the colon, unable to produce the vigorous contraction needed for defæcation, distends to accommodate the collection of fermenting fæces.

4. *Want of Training in Regular Habits, or Stress of Circumstances of Daily Life.* A child should be taught very early the habit of defæcation at a definite daily time. Usually after breakfast is the best time, when the loading of the stomach with foods sets up a reflex strong wave of peristalsis in the colon,

Exercise. Exercise is essential for health. Without it, the vital processes slow down, waste products accumulate, muscles lose tone, and metabolism is lowered. The results of exercise may be summarized thus:

1. **Muscles develop and muscle tone is improved.**
2. Fuel food is needed for combustion, therefore **appetite is stimulated.**
3. Oxygen is needed for combustion and the carbon dioxide produced has to be expelled, therefore **respiration is stimulated and deepened.**
4. The muscles are in constant movement so that **lymph and blood circulations are quickened.**
5. Peristalsis is increased and **constipation avoided.**
6. **Improved circulation clears the organs of waste products,** which are excreted via the kidneys and skin.
7. This increase of blood supply to the organs greatly **improves general metabolism.**
8. **The mind is stimulated** by a feeling of fitness.

The best forms of exercise are those which use all groups of muscles equally, such as walking, swimming, and dancing. Overstrain must be avoided, because this is liable to affect the heart.

Muscle Fatigue. This occurs after violent or prolonged working of muscles. The muscles are unable to respond to nerve messages. Lactic acid has accumulated because oxygen was not taken in fast enough, and rest is necessary until sufficient oxygen has been taken in to achieve the removal of the lactic acid from the tissues. Rest, heat and rubbing will restore the muscles.

Rest, Sleep and Recreation. Fatigue is of two kinds. One is *fatigue of muscles* (already discussed), and the other, *fatigue of the brain and nervous system,* occurs rhythmically in every twenty-four hours when, the body having been placed in a position of repose, consciousness is lost, and the brain rests. If the body is forced to continue acting in acute fatigue, the brain will "go to sleep" while the muscles continue to contract in such reflex actions as walking, but actions that require super-vision of the intellect cannot be carried out.

This brain fatigue and sleep rhythm is natural, but there are other and worse causes of brain fatigue such as worry, anxiety and strain, and sleep is not restful while these persist.

The amount of sleep needed varies greatly from the twenty or more hours for the baby to the five or six hours' sleep of some people in later life.

The conditions that induce restful sleep are a quiet room; darkness; a bed, with a comfortable mattress, preferably spring-interior or latex-foam; bedclothes that are sufficiently warm but also light; night clothes that are comfortable and loose; fresh air without chill; and complete relaxation of all muscles. Heavy meals should not be taken just before going to bed, but a hot drink after a warm bath is often helpful. Most import-ant of all is a mind at peace; worry and concentration will certainly hinder sleep and cause a weariness in the morning.

Recreation may be physical or mental and should be both. The mind, to be rested and refreshed, should be switched away from its usual work and preoccupations on to some quite different subject which must be of real interest. Hobbies often provide such recreation.

Fresh Air and Sunlight. These have a double beneficial action; they stimulate the mind and they produce impor-tant effects on the skin which result in general improvement of body metabolism.

Fresh air moving over the skin evaporates sweat and cools the body in hot weather. It stimulates circulation in the skin blood vessels, ensures good ventilation of the lungs, and helps to produce restful sleep.

4*

Sunlight has many effects on the body; some of these are:

1. Infra-red rays are felt as heat.

2. Erythema follows, and later pigmentation in the cells of the epidermis, produced by the ultra-violet rays. This "sunburn" is Nature's protection against the further action of infra-red rays, with possible heat-stroke.

3. Ultra-violet rays act on cholesterol and other sterols in the sebum on the skin surface and produce vitamin D (calciferol) which enables the blood to carry calcium and phosphorus.

4. Endocrine glands are affected; the thyroid for instance, is stimulated.

5. Bacteria are destroyed, more by increase of anti-bodies and leucocytes in the blood than by direct action of rays.

6. The mind and body are stimulated; better appetite and sleep and general feeling of fitness should result.

3. Habits and Mental Outlook

Training in good habits both physical and mental profoundly affects the life of the individual and should be started very early.

Physical habits such as the daily bath, teeth cleaning, nose breathing, daily bowel action, and punctual regular sleep, are begun in babyhood.

Mental habits are of incalculable importance. Bad ones can work havoc in life, while good ones are of untold value. They begin in the earliest days, for good or for ill, and grow with the child. Examples, of such habits, good and bad, are obedience, discipline, grumbling, cheerfulness, observation, concentration, unselfishness. Bad habits of mind, so easily acquired in early years, are extremely difficult to eradicate in later life.

CHAPTER VII

HYGIENE OF THE FAMILY AT ALL AGES

The Baby

DURING the first fourteen days of life the baby is under the supervision of the midwife. After that the mother should take him regularly to the Infant Welfare Clinic. The health visitor who is present at the clinics also visits in the home to give any further help and advice.

Feeding. Normally the baby will be breast fed, probably four-hourly, with the first feed at 6 or 7 a.m. and the last at 10 or 11 p.m. He should be dry and warm when fed, and should rest once or twice during a feed, and if he sleeps well, has a rising weight curve and is not fretful, it will be clear that he is having enough. A little boiled water may be given from a teaspoon if he is thirsty. The mother needs a good nourishing diet meanwhile, of the same type as the antenatal diet. Supplementary feeds should be given only by doctor's orders.

Artificial Feeding. This, if necessary, will be given according to the doctor's orders. Modified cow's milk may be used or one of the brands of dried milk.

Great care must be taken in the preparation of feeds in order to avoid contamination and the mother will be shown how to do this, and how to avoid touching the teat except by the rim and how to hold the bottle. After the feed the bottle is washed first in cold water, then in hot soapy water with the aid of a brush. The teat is turned inside out, and is washed in the same way and rubbed with salt. Both are rinsed and are either boiled and kept covered in the same water or are kept covered in a solution of Milton. Alternatively, the teats may be kept dry in a special container.

Milk should never be left uncovered so that flies can contaminate it, thus causing the spread of gastro-enteritis and other diseases. It should be kept covered and in a safe that is fly-proof and as cool as possible. Dried milks are quite safe.

Babies require 50 calories per lb. of their weight, per day, and milk gives 20 calories for 1 oz. The temperature of feeds should be 100° F. and times of feeding should be as for breast feeding. One tablespoonful of concentrated orange juice and one teaspoonful of cod liver oil should be given daily.

Weaning and Mixed Feeding. This usually starts in the fifth or sixth month. Gradually breast milk is replaced by cow's milk and thickened feeds are added, Farex, groats, vegetable broth, custard, rusks to chew and later sieved fruit and vegetables, steamed fish, minced meat, potato and butter. Fruit juice is given daily and cod- or halibut-liver oil.

Toilet. A small baby should be bathed in a warm room with the window closed. The temperature of the water should be 100° F., and the soap used should be a pure baby soap. When all is ready, the mother or nurse washes her hands well, and then, taking the baby on her knees, washes first his face, using only clean water, and wool. The eyes are sponged with damp wool, and the nose should be left untouched if possible, and the mouth is not cleaned, since the lining mucous membrane is very delicate. The scalp is then washed (using soap) and dried. The napkin is now removed, the body is washed all over, the baby lifted into the bath, held carefully, and well rinsed. He is then lifted back on to the knees, covered with a soft towel, dabbed thoroughly dry, and powdered with a good baby powder.

Clothes. The wool of which baby clothes are made should be soft and non-irritating since the skin is very sensitive. Garments should be few but sufficiently warm, and never tight or constricting. The head should not be covered, but must be shaded from strong sunlight.

Napkins must be very soft; a Harrington's square is best. They must be changed whenever wet, washed with soap that does not contain soda, boiled and dried.

Sleep. A baby up to one month old should be sleeping all the time he is not feeding or being bathed and dressed. From 10 p.m. to 6 a.m. his sleep should be uninterrupted. If it is not, the cause (if he is healthy) may be cold, overheating, a stuffy room, discomfort due to wet clothing, over-feeding, or he may have been allowed to form a habit of expecting too much attention. After the last feed he should neither be picked up, talked to nor rocked, and he will then quickly form the "sleep habit".

The room should never be stuffy; windows should be open top and bottom and the baby kept sufficiently (but not excessively) warm in his cot. The mattress should be firm and the coverings should be light and kept fresh and well aired. Needless to say, a baby should never sleep in the mother's bed.

In summer he may sleep much of the day out of doors, his head being shaded from direct sunlight.

Stools. These should be soft and yellow, with no curds, and there should be three or four a day. A baby should be trained from his earliest days to pass urine and fæces by holding him, after feeding, over a babies' training chamber, the baby and chamber being supported on the lap.

Weight. The baby should be weighed weekly and the weight chart should show in two weeks his birth weight regained after a slight loss, and thereafter a gain of 5 or 6 oz. a week. The rate slows down a little after six months, and at one year he should have trebled his birth weight.

Teeth. About the sixth month the teeth begin to come through, beginning with the two incisors in the lower jaw, then the upper incisors, and soon after one year the premolars. On no account may "dummies" be given to suck with the idea of helping the process.

Exercise. Babies should be allowed to lie on a blanket and kick for a time each day, after they are a few weeks old. They should have washable bright coloured toys, and soft toys to cuddle. Later they may be put in a playpen, in the garden when possible, where they can exercise their muscles and be safe from harm. They should not be encouraged to walk too soon.

Habits. It is never too young to begin training. Good habits of sleep and bowel action have been mentioned, and are easily acquired. Everything should be done punctually and quietly. Those who look after babies should not be erratic or "nervy", and a calm, happy atmosphere should surround them from earliest days. They must feel a sense of love and security. Any lack of confidence and affection will react on their nervous systems with grave consequences.

Children from One to Five Years

During these years the child is growing and developing rapidly both mentally and physically and his environment is of the utmost importance. The child in a happy home of whatever station in life has the first essentials for sound development. He feels no insecurity. he is loved and cared for, fed and clothed and his mother provides for all his needs. If this normal life is not possible due to the mother's daily outside work, the day nurseries will give the child skilled care and training until he is fetched by his mother in the evening.

The Toilet. The daily warm bath should be a routine wherever possible. In homes where this cannot be managed a warm sponging should take its place. The child will be taught to wash and dry himself and clean his teeth, using his own tooth brush, face cloth and towels. He learns gradually to brush and comb his hair and to dress himself.

Meals. These should be three a day. On waking he should have the juice of an orange in a little water, and his meals would be of the following type:

Breakfast.	Dinner.	Tea.
Porridge and milk or other cereal. Milk. Egg, bacon or fish. Toast and butter.	A little meat, fish, chicken or rabbit well cut up. Potato, a little green or other vegetables well cut up. Fruit, stewed or fresh, with milk pudding or custard, or steamed pudding and fresh fruit. Water to drink.	Milk 6–10 oz. Brown bread or rusks with butter and honey or jam. Fruit, fresh or stewed, with custard or junket.
Mid-morning		**Supper 6–6.30**
Milk.		Milk.

He should not be allowed sweets between meals, but just after them if wanted. He should never have sweets in bed after the teeth cleaning is done, unless a drink of water or a piece of apple is given afterwards, since the acid produced by fermenting sugar destroys the enamel of the teeth.

Clothes. These should be as few and as simple as possible, and they should be loose. They should be made of aertex, silk and wool or wool, thin in summer and thick in winter, since these materials absorb perspiration and are bad conductors of heat. Vest and pants under the jumper suit or tunic are enough for a boy, and vest and panties for a girl. Arms, legs and neck should be bare in summer. Jumpers, pullovers, cardigans and warm but light-weight overcoats are added as required.

Pyjamas are worn at night, the thickness varying with the seasons.

Shoes should have good soles, but should not be too heavy, and must never cramp the feet.

Bowels. Plenty of water to drink; fruit and vegetables, brown bread and porridge in the diet; exercise, and training, are all means towards the forming of a regular habit by which the colon is emptied each day after breakfast. Nothing should interfere with this daily habit, and if necessary syrup of figs or senna or some other mild aperient should be given.

Sleep. All small children need at least 12 hours' sleep in 24 hours. All should have a sleep period during the day, but the length of time varies with the age and type of child. If the rest can be taken in the fresh air it is a very good arrangement.

Exercise and Play. Playtimes are a most important part of the child's daily life. There is no need for expensive toys. Anything with which the child can construct and experiment will serve, and children prefer to make their own games and use their imagination. As much as possible of their play should be out of doors. As they grow older and want to climb, swings, rope ladders, etc., should be provided for them.

Training. The years of the toddler are the great training time of his life, and the subject is too wide for discussion here.

The habits formed at this time will persist in some form or other through his life, and those who have charge of him should regard the training of his character as of the first importance.

Little children believe implicitly everything that is said to them, and it is a sad thing for the "grown-up" through whom they first learn not to do so. The small child is always curious, and his questions should be encouraged and answered with truth.

The two extremes of constant suppression and inordinate praise are equally tragedies for a child.

He should begin to learn self-control from baby days, and also obedience, which will never be taught by scolding.

He should learn early to do things for himself and to be helpful and resourceful. In the words of The Education Act—"The aim of the new concept of education is to educate the child according to his age, aptitude and ability."

The School Child

School years are a time of rapid growth and development and the secondary school education of today (see p. 251) takes a wide view of the needs, both mental and physical, of the school child. He must be trained to realize that he is a member of a youthful company in which he is expected to play his part and contribute to the general welfare. He learns from small beginnings to take responsibility, and under wise direction to develop his individuality in his social environment.

The aim of the new concept of education is to discover the child's chief interest and to focus his training mainly on that subject so that he may become proficient in his chosen occupation, whether languages, science, art, commercial or other subject. Meanwhile the basic general education, which he received up to eleven years, is continued and correlated with his chosen work.

Physical training in a properly equipped gymnasium, swimming, and outdoor games of all kinds in playing fields, with inter-school matches, are all included in the secondary school curriculum, all equipment being provided by the Local Authorities.

In the classroom great attention is paid to ventilation, lighting, correct height of desks and chairs and the child's posture. (See illustration on p. 259.)

Health. This is under constant supervision. Medical and dental examinations, inspections by the school nurse, free milk and good dinners at low cost all safeguard the physical well-being of the children.

Out-of-school activities that will contribute to the spirit of fellowship are provided and encouraged. Orchestras, dramatic clubs, and notably camping—all these and many other varieties of spare time activities contribute in a real sense to a child's education.

Camping

Camping, apart from its special appeal as a great adventure, has a real value. The open air life (especially for city children), the comradeship, camp routine, duties and discipline, the nature study, map reading, exploring and many other activities all contribute new interests, and not least the gatherings round the camp fire at night.

The Hygiene of the Camp.

Latrines. These are sited at least 50–100 yards from buildings or wells. Cubicles are constructed with poles and sacking, allowing one cubicle to five or six girls or boys. Long narrow slit trenches are dug about 18 inches deep. The earth removed is piled up at the end of the trench, where a small shovel is placed for throwing earth over the excreta. A toilet roll is provided in an improvised container, *e.g.* an Ovaltine tin. Some guide companies improvise seats with packing cases. A sanitary patrol goes round each morning and evening inspecting and disinfecting. Outside the cubicles there is a stand with washbowl, soap and towels.

Water Supply. This must be near at hand; water for drinking and cooking must be pure and safe; for washing, well or spring water and sometimes water from a stream may be used.

Washing Facilities. These may be planned in the same type of cubicle, in girls' camps, the basins being raised on improvised stands. River water may be used for washing, but not for cleaning the teeth. Soapy water may be thrown into a ditch or a dry soakage pit, but not into a pond or stream where animals drink.

Food Storage. The food tent should be in the shade. Improvised cupboards for different types of food can be made by using wooden packing cases placed on their sides and raised off the ground. Muslin is used for fly-proof coverings. Milk bottles and bowls containing butter and margarine should be covered with muslin and stand in large bowls of water into which the muslin dips. Meat should be fetched from the butcher daily. Pails of drinking water should be covered with muslin. Larders may be improvised as shown in the illustration.

Washing-up. All scraps should be put into a covered pail except tea leaves, egg shells, and fruit stones, which should be burned. Arrangements may be made for disposing of the food waste at a farm. Greasy water is poured through a sieve lined with grass into a suitable ditch or dug hole. The greasy grass is burned. A deep hole is dug for a refuse pit and when camp is struck this is filled in with earth.

A Salvage Sack. This should always be provided and be hung in a sheltered place.

An Incinerator. This may be built with old bricks and used for burning kitchen waste.

The First Aid Tent. This contains a camp bed, blankets, hot water bottle, thermometer, medicine glass, dressings, bandages, scissors and other necessities, as well as simple first aid remedies. The names, addresses

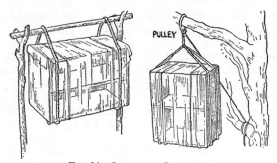

FIG. 34.—IMPROVISED LARDERS.
These are made from Orange Boxes completely covered with
Muslin, which is kept in place with Elastic Tapes.

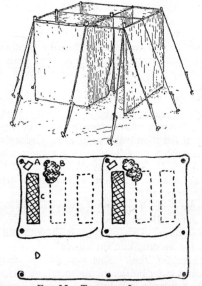

FIG. 35.—TWO-UNIT LATRINE.
A. Paper; B. Earth and Shovel; C. Trench; D. Passage.
From Organised Camping *by permission of the Controller of H.M.
Stationery Office.*

and telephone numbers of the nearest doctors should be hung in a prominent place.

Personal kit required:

    Shorts and skirts.
or Blouses or jumpers and skirt;
or Uniform.
    Mackintosh with hood.
    Wind jacket or cardigan.
    Gum boots.
    Walking shoes—2 pairs.
    Canvas shoes.
    Socks or stockings—several pairs.
    Warm pyjamas.
    Change of underclothing.
    Handkerchiefs.
    Mending materials.

  Also:

    Toothbrush and paste, nailbrush, hairbrush and comb, face cloth, coat hanger, shoe polish, knife, fork and spoon, 2 mugs, 2 plates, torch, pillow and mirror.

Bedding. Four blankets are needed and must be arranged to go under as well as over the sleeping bag. These should be aired daily, and if they are damp, arrangements must be made to dry them and also any damp clothes.

The many other details of camp life cannot be included here.

The Worker

See "Occupational Health", Chapter XV.

Old Age

The change in the way of life for old people is conditioned by various factors, some sudden, some gradual. Retirement from their work brings to some welcome opportunities to enjoy more fully their spare-time recreations; others find it hard to compensate for the loss of the interests of their working life, and for them adjustment is difficult.

Physical changes, due to the slowing down of body metabolism, are gradual and call for modifications in diet and exercise. As age advances the blood pressure rises and, although some daily exercise is necessary, it should not be so strenuous as to overtax the heart. More rest and sleep are needed, but old people vary in the amount they require.

The diet is gradually adjusted to the lessened needs of the body. Fat tends to be deposited in many people if too much carbohydrate food is eaten, since only small quantities are needed for muscle activity, the excess being converted into fat. For this reason less starchy foods as well as fats should be included in the diet.

Because the body tissues need less renewing, protein should be taken in smaller quantities, and in the very old it should be of an easily digestible type. In these ways the total calorie intake is suitably reduced.

In general, old people should have what they like to eat as far as possible, unless their wishes are unwise on account of disease. They should not take a heavy meal at night, nor too large a meal at any time, and usually the stimulant they are used to, taken in reason, is good for them.

The Mind. The contribution that a nurse can make towards the happiness of the old depends on her own personality, which is far more important in this case (unless the patient is acutely ill) than the amount of training she has had or the knowledge she possesses.

Old people have no longer the power to be adaptable, and if the nurse will be considerate of their likes and dislikes they will usually respond with gratitude out of all proportion to the nurse's effort.

(See also Chapter XV.)

CHAPTER VIII

CLOTHING AND FABRICS

Regulation of Body Temperature

THE various fabrics used for clothing play a large part in assisting the heat-regulating mechanism of the body to maintain the temperature within normal limits. Temperature balance is carefully adjusted in the following way:

(a) When air temperature is cold, skin blood vessels contract in order to limit radiation of heat, sweat production is at a minimum, exercise of muscles is encouraged to produce heat (failing voluntary exercise, shivering occurs).

(b) When air temperature is hot, skin blood vessels dilate to increase radiation, sweat production is enormously increased to cool the body by evaporation, exercise is avoided as far as possible.

Clothes form an envelope round the body which either assists the sweat to evaporate and conducts the heat away, so allowing cooling to take place, or retains both heat and moisture, so helping to keep the body warm. The points of importance when considering material and clothes with regard to hygiene are:

1. To what extent they retain heat or conduct it away.
2. To what extent they absorb moisture (sweat) or allow it to evaporate.
3. Looseness or tightness.
4. Weight.
5. Colour.
6. Origin of materials and other points.

1 and **2. Conduction and Absorption.** From a health point of view this is the most important consideration. The air next to the skin receives from it heat and moisture, and the fibres of the clothing material either keep this in or let it emerge. To take two examples:

(1) *Wool*. Its fibres contain grease, do not easily absorb moisture, and among the fibres is much air which holds the moisture and is a bad conductor of heat. It therefore keeps heat in (unless so loosely woven that the wind penetrates), and is a "warm material".

(2) *Linen*. Its fibres absorb from the skin the moisture secreted, which then passes off into the air, carrying heat with it. It is then a good conductor of heat and a "cool material".

Fabrics

In order of *heat and moisture retaining*.	In order of *heat conducting and evaporation of moisture*.
Plastic.	Linen.
Fur.	Cotton.
Leather.	Artificial silk.
Wool.	Silk.
Silk.	Wool.
Artificial silk.	Leather.
Cotton.	Fur.
Linen.	Plastic.

3. Looseness. Clothes should be loose enough to allow a layer of air next to the skin, and any real constriction is bad. Children especially should wear loose garments, which should hang from the shoulders, leaving legs and arms bare.

In tropical countries tight clothing is dangerous

because it prevents heat from the body escaping, and heat stroke results.

4. Weight. This is not synonymous with warmth. Clothing should be light.

5. Colour. Dark colours, especially red and black, absorb some of the heat rays (infra-red), while light colours do not. Dark clothes are therefore warmer.

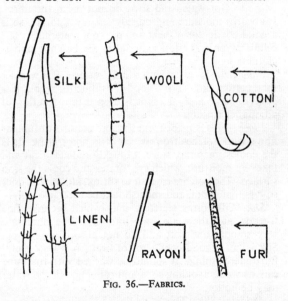

FIG. 36.—FABRICS.

6. Various Fabrics. *Wool,* from skins of animals, varies greatly. Its fibres are tubes made of tiny overlapping scales. They contain natural fat, so do not absorb moisture readily, and much air, which is a bad conductor of heat, is held among them. Wool is warm, but for undergarments is apt to irritate the skin.

Wool shrinks and becomes harsh when washed with

very hot water or with soda or any other alkali or bleaching substance, because the oil is removed from its fibres and the little scales harden. It should be washed in warm, soft water with superfatted soap, dried only in moderate heat, and ironed with a damp cloth.

Cotton. This is made from fibres from the covering of cotton plant seeds. The tubes are flattened and twisted. Hot water and soda do not harm the fibres. It absorbs moisture and quickly lets it evaporate, so is a good conductor of heat and a "cool material". The cellular type of cotton material is the best for underclothing.

Flannelette is cotton with a fluffy surface. It is warmer than cotton, but is not a good substitute for wool. It is easily inflammable unless it is dipped in a solution of alum after rinsing.

Linen. This is made from flax and consists of tubular fibres with notches from which little fibres grow. It is the coolest material, since it quickly radiates heat and takes up moisture, which evaporates and cools the skin surface. The notches cause it to shrink, although it does so less than wool, and soda should be used sparingly.

Silk. Silkworms secrete a fluid which becomes fine threads, and these are spun into silk. The fibres are very smooth and soft and do not absorb water well. Silk is not a good conductor of heat, so is very useful for underclothing. It should be washed with the same care as wool, avoiding soda and rubbing, but the water may be hotter.

Artificial Silk. This is made from cellulose of trees and plants. The fibres are neither so strong nor so light as silk. It does not absorb moisture well and it conducts heat readily, so is not a warm fabric. It is inexpensive, and is very extensively used for underclothing.

Nylon is a synthetic material obtained from coal tar.

Leather and Fur. These are the warmest clothing possible. Leather is wind-proof, and lined with wool and closed at ankles, wrists and neck it is used for very cold climates.

Waterproof Material. This is fabric treated with chemicals or impregnated with quick-drying oils.

Plastic is obtained from coal tar.

Conclusion. Underclothes of silk, wool, silk and wool, cellular cotton, artificial silk, wool and cotton all have their merits with regard to climate and cost.

Constricting garments should be avoided, especially for children.

Sun and air should have access to the skin to a reasonable extent.

CHAPTER IX

INFECTION AND DISINFECTION
HYGIENE OF THE WARD AND SICK ROOM

INFECTION

WHEN bacteria gain entrance to the body and grow and multiply in the tissues, the condition is spoken of as *infection*.

Bacteria, or micro-organisms, are minute unicellular organisms. The cell consists of protoplasm with a nucleus and an outer membrane or cell wall.

They live, reproduce and die in earth, water, vegetation, on and in the bodies of men and animals, alive or dead, and in culture media in the laboratory.

The conditions they require for life and growth vary greatly.

Their food is obtained from the surrounding medium, in solution in water, and consists of protein, carbohydrate and mineral salts. These they absorb from the fluid which passes through their cell wall. If deprived of moisture and food they die, usually quickly, though a few varieties can continue to live for some time.

Oxygen they need, but not all are able to take it from the air.

Aerobes are those that need air to obtain their oxygen.

Anaerobes are those that cannot live in the presence of air.

Facultative organisms are those that can exist under either condition.

Temperature. Most bacteria grow well at a temperature between 98° and 100° F. Below 50° F. and above 110° F. they cease to grow. At 160° F. most kinds die, and boiling water kills all except the sporing types. Low temperatures are not so fatal, since many kinds of organisms are able to revive when conditions become warmer.

The *reaction* of their surroundings is very important to bacteria. Most of them like a neutral or slightly alkaline reaction, but each variety has its special preference, and any change in the acidity or alkalinity of its surroundings will stop its growth.

Reproduction. This is by division or fission, and is very rapid unless it is checked by unfavourable surroundings.

Spores. Some bacteria of the rod-shaped type (bacilli) in unfavourable circumstances are able to form themselves into a resistant phase or "spore". In this phase they can resist drying, heat to some extent, cold and disinfectants. When circumstances are favourable again, the bacillus resumes its ordinary or "vegetative" phase, and proceeds to multiply and manufacture its various products.

Examples are the bacilli of tetanus and anthrax, and various bacilli that cause putrefaction.

The work done by bacteria is of vital importance. Their good works keep the earth habitable; their bad works are only too well known.

Putrefaction. This is the breaking up, by bacteria called *saprophytes*, of dead organic matter, both animal and vegetable, into nitrogenous salts, water, and gases with unpleasant odours. These changes are achieved by means of enzymes or ferments, produced by the organisms, which act on the material in much the same way as digestive enzymes in the body.

Fermentation. This is produced in organic substances by many kinds of bacteria, and the chemical changes result in the production of gases and acids. Fermenting of wine and souring of milk are two examples.

Nitrification. This work of bacteria is essential for the life of plants, and therefore for animal life on the earth. Plants need nitrogen, and they cannot obtain it from the air; they must therefore take it from the soil, in the form of salts (nitrates and nitrites) in solution. These salts are produced in the soil by the work of nitrifying bacteria from urea and ammonia, substances which are present due to the action of saprophytic bacteria on dead organic matter.

Yet other organisms, nitrogen-fixation bacteria, are able to take nitrogen from the air, and entering the root tubercles of certain plants, peas, beans, etc., they convert it into nitrates for plant use.

Disease Production. When the substances produced by bacteria are poisonous to living tissues, they are spoken of as *toxins*, and the bacteria as *pathogenic*. If these poisons pass out of the organisms and spread in the tissues they are called *exotoxins*. If, however, the poison formed remains in the bacteria it is an *endotoxin*, set free only on the death of the organisms. Pathogenic bacteria are parasites, since they live on, and receive their nourishment from, another living organism (their host).

Classification. Bacteria are classified according to their shapes as:

1. *Cocci*—round cells, found in:

        (*a*) Groups—staphylococci.
        (*b*) Chains—streptococci.
        (*c*) Pairs—diplococci.

2. *Bacilli*—rod-shaped, *e.g.* tubercle bacilli, typhoid bacilli.

Some of these form spores.

3. *Spirilla and vibrios*—curved, wavy, or comma-shaped rods, *e.g.* the vibrio of cholera.

Spirilla.   Vibrios.

4. *Spirochætes*—wavy organisms that move with undulating movements, *e.g.* the *Spirochæta pallida* (now called *Treponema pallidum*) of syphilis.

5. *Protozoa*—belonging to the lowest scale of the

animal kingdom. They are unicellular animals, *e.g.* the amœba of dysentery.

6. *Filterable viruses*—organisms too small to be seen under most microscopes. They can pass through a porcelain filter, *e.g.* the organisms of measles, mumps, chickenpox, smallpox, influenza, etc.

Explanation of Certain Terms

Specific Disease. One caused by a special organism peculiar to that disease, *e.g.* diphtheria, tuberculosis.

Incubation. The time between the entry of the bacteria and the onset of symptoms. The organisms have been developing and multiplying meanwhile.

Contacts. Those who have been with an infected person and who, themselves, may or may not have become infected.

Quarantine Period. The time necessary to keep contacts isolated—*i.e.*, the longest time that can elapse before the symptoms (of the disease in question) appear.

Sporadic. Scattered or isolated cases of a disease.

Epidemic. Rapid spread of an infectious disease. It dies down in time, leaving the people with improved immunity.

Pandemic. An epidemic which spreads over all the world.

Endemic. A disease always present in a certain district.

Immunity. The power possessed by a person's blood and tissues to resist any particular disease. He may have sufficient resistance at birth, or he may acquire it (*a*) by having an attack of the disease, or (*b*) by repeated injections of vaccines (preparations of the organism of the disease). He may be made *temporarily* immune by injections of serum from the blood of an immune person or animal. (See Chapter XVI, p. 277).

Fomites. Any articles that have been near enough to an infectious patient to be contaminated with bacteria—*e.g.*, books, linen, furniture, etc.

Carriers. Those who carry the organisms of a disease in their bodies and discharge them, so becoming a danger to others. They may be:

1. Contact carriers:

(*a*) A person who is in the incubation period of a disease.

(*b*) A person who has not had the disease, but has come into contact with the organism and is carrying and discharging it.

2. Convalescent:

(*a*) Temporary; (*b*) Chronic; a person who has recovered from the disease, but who is still carrying and discharging the organism.

Notification

Infectious diseases must be notified to the Medical Officer of Health, and the notifications are sent up by him each week to the Ministry of Health.

Notifiable Diseases

Smallpox.

Cholera.

Diphtheria.

Scarlet fever.

Enteric fever (typhoid and paratyphoid).

Dysentery (amœbic and bacillary).

Typhus fever.

Puerperal fever and puerperal pyrexia.

Continued fever.

Relapsing fever.

Erysipelas.

Plague.

Acute primary pneumonia.

Acute influenzal pneumonia.

Encephalitis lethargica.

Acute poliomyelitis.

Cerebrospinal meningitis.

Malaria.

Ophthalmia neonatorum.

Tuberculosis.

The Minister of Health, or the Local Authority with his consent, may make other diseases notifiable at any time. Measles, chickenpox and acute rheumatism are examples.

Anthrax is notifiable to the Chief Inspector of Factories, and some diseases of animals to the local M.O.H.

Methods by Which Communicable Diseases may Spread.

Method.	Diseases
1. Droplet Infection. Bacteria sprayed out on droplets of secretions from nose and throat in sneezing, coughing and even breathing and talking.	Diphtheria, measles, scarlet fever, mumps, influenza, cerebrospinal meningitis, whooping-cough, anterior polio-myclitis.
2. Water. Contaminated with excreta.	Typhoid fever, dysentery, cholera.
3. Milk. (a) From the cow.	Tuberculosis, sore throat, abortus infection.
(b) Contaminated by milkers, water, flies, dust.	Typhoid fever, diphtheria, scarlet fever, infantile diarrhœa, food poisoning.
4. Carriers.	Typhoid fever, diphtheria, cerebrospinal fever, dysentery, anterior poliomyelitis.
5. Flies.	Many infectious diseases, especially typhoid, dysentery, infantile diarrhœa, cholera, food poisoning.
6. Parasites. (a) *Fleas.*	(a) Rat fleas carry plague.

Methods by which Communicable Diseases may Spread—*Continued*

Method.	Diseases.

6. **Parasites—***Continued*
   (b) *Lice.*
   (c) *Bugs.*
 	
   (d) *Mites.*
	(b)
	&
	(c) — Bites of these insects provide a channel for entry of infection—*e.g.*, typhus fever.
	(d) African tick fever.

7. **Dust.** Bacteria that can live when dried.	Tuberculosis, anthrax, streptococcal infections.
8. **Food.** (a) Infected through water contaminated by sewage.	Typhoid Dysentery Cholera — By oysters, watercress, and any fruit or vegetables washed in contaminated water.
(b) Contaminated by hands or flies.	Typhoid, dysentery, infantile diarrhœa, food poisoning.
9. **Sputum.** Also fomites contaminated by it.	Tuberculosis of lung, influenzal and acute pneumonia.
10. **Mosquitoes.**	Malaria, yellow fever.
11. **Secretions from lesions.**	Smallpox—secretions and scabs. Chickenpox — secretions and scabs. Syphilis. Gonorrhœa. Ophthalmia neonatorum.
12. **Direct contact.**	Any infectious disease.

Methods of Destroying Bacteria or Preventing Their Growth

1. Fresh Air and Wind. By their drying power and by access of oxygen to the organisms.

2. Sunlight. By ultra-violet rays.

3. Cold. Cold storage and refrigerators are used for preserving food. (Note that the typhoid bacillus can live in ice.)

4. Dehydration. Used in preserving foods, since it removes the moisture necessary for bacterial growth.

5. Heat. (*a*) *Boiling* kills all bacteria and, if sufficiently prolonged, kills spores.

(*b*) *Steam Disinfection by Steam under Pressure.* Flowing steam (from boiling water) has a temperature of 212° F. Steam as used in disinfectors is under a pressure of about 15 lbs. (to the square inch), which raises the temperature to about 250° F. It penetrates into mattresses, blankets, dressing drums, etc., and gives up its heat as it condenses into water. It is all this liberated heat that kills bacteria. The Washington-Lyons steam disinfector is a large chamber surrounded by a hollow jacket, with a door at each end, opening into different rooms, the "infected" and the "disinfected" sides. Infected articles are put in a wire cradle that runs on rails. This is pushed in and the heavy doors securely fastened. Steam from a boiler is passed into the hollow surrounding jacket to warm up the walls, and then some of the air in the chamber is drawn out to leave a partial vacuum. Steam is then admitted to the chamber (the vacuum sucking it in) and maintained at a sufficient pressure for twenty minutes. At the end the vacuum pipe is used to suck out the steam, and yet again to suck in air to dry the articles. This air is filtered and heated so that it is sterile in sterilizers for dressing drums.

The wire cradle is then drawn out at the "disinfected" end. Temperature, pressure and time are recorded on a graph.

(c) *Disinfection.* A method without steam is necessary for bedding including spring-interior and latex-foam mattresses, clothing, rubber goods, toys, papers, etc.

For this purpose a disinfectant vapour is used, either in a special disinfector, or by means of a vaporizer attached to the steam disinfector.

This is filled with the disinfectant fluid which when heated vaporizes, the vapour being sucked into the chamber. At the end of the required time exhaust fans are switched on and the fumes are drawn out to atmosphere. No steam is used.

(d) *Hot Air.* Small hot air "ovens" are used to sterilize glassware in laboratories. The temperature is higher than is necessary in steam disinfection.

(e) *Burning.* This is useful for infected articles of little value—*e.g.* papers, infected dressings.

6. Disinfectants.   Chemical substances that kill bacteria. In a weaker solution they may prevent their growth and are then called *antiseptics*.

NOTE. Deodorants are substances that mask unpleasant odours. They do not kill bacteria.

DISINFECTION

Methods in Use

Recommendations have been made by the Medical Research Council for methods of disinfection.

Much use is made of "black" and "white" fluid.

Black fluid is a crude coal tar preparation which is diluted according to the purpose for which it is to be used.

The formula of white fluid is:

> Borax   1·5
> Formalin 2·5
> Phenol   0·4
> add water up to 100 parts.

The following are methods in use:

Mattresses. Hair and spring-interior mattresses may be steam disinfected.

For Latex foam or Sorbo mattresses steam disinfection cannot be used. If no other method is available, the cover is removed and cleaned in disinfectant solution, and the interior is sponged with weak disinfectant (*e.g.* lysol, 1 in 40), rinsed and dried in the air but not in sunlight. Rubber mattresses, as well as all other types, can be disinfected in a vapour disinfector.

Blankets and Pillows. These are sent for either steam or vapour disinfection.

Linen. This is received at the bedside into a special bin containing disinfectant (*e.g.* lysol, 1 in 80, or white fluid) and covered with a lid. The linen soaks in this solution for 12 hours and may then be sent to the laundry in a special marked bag.

Crockery and Cutlery. All articles should be boiled for 5 minutes.

Excreta. In cases of infection of the intestinal tract excreta should be mixed with an equal quantity of a 1 in 10 solution of an effective general disinfectant (*e.g.* black or white fluid) and stand for two hours before disposal.

Bedpans. These if not steam sterilized may be boiled or immersed in a 1 in 80 solution of a general disinfectant of the black or white fluid type for at least one hour. They are then washed and dried.

Refuse and Waste Water. A covered pail containing a 1 in 10 solution of disinfectant (black or white fluid) is needed to receive refuse awaiting disposal.

Sputum Containers. In hospital wards cartons are collected daily or if necessary twice a day, and are burned in an incinerator. In sanatoria cartons in metal frames are often used. The patient places the carton on a tray that is carried round by a porter wearing gown, mask and gloves. From the tray the cartons are tilted into the incinerator so that no one but the patient handles them. The metal frames, collected separately, are sterilized with the metal trays.

The Infected Room or Premises

Rooms are not normally disinfected (except for vermin). Great stress is laid on current disinfection and prevention of cross-infection. Terminal disinfection is limited to steam disinfection of bedding and thorough airing and cleaning.

Disinfection of Verminous Premises.

(1) *Formalin.* A 2 per cent. solution is sprayed over the entire room and contents. Alternatively, paraform tablets (30 for a medium sized room) are vaporized over a spirit lamp. The room is sealed for 24 hours.

(2) *Hydrocyanic Acid Gas.* This is highly dangerous but very efficient for exterminating insects, rats and other pests. It is much used for ridding ships of rats. For houses it is extremely dangerous and must be used only by experts. It is expelled into a sealed room from cylinders.

Nursing an Infectious Patient in a Private House

Current Disinfection.

The Room. There is probably no choice of room, as the patient will be already in bed. Objects and furniture not needed for use or comfort should be removed. They must be disinfected.

Cleaning. Raising and scattering dust is to be

avoided. Damp dusting, vacuum cleaning and polishing are all good methods. The dust should be burned.

Fire. A coal fire, if available, is useful for burning infective material, dust, food remains, etc. Gas and electric fires require special care with regard to ventilation.

Linen. This is treated as explained on page 133.

Crockery. This is washed and kept separate in or near the room and must not be sent to the kitchen.

Food. Remaining food must not be returned to the kitchen. Any waste is disposed of in the refuse bin or burnt.

Bedpans and Excreta. These, in cases of intestinal infection, need special treatment. A lavatory should be reserved if possible. If this cannot be managed great care should be taken to disinfect thoroughly. Bedpans and excreta should be treated as described on page 133.

Disinfecting-table. This stands at the entrance to the room, unless there is a reserved bathroom. It is set with water, soap, nailbrush, hand lotion and towel.

Gowns and Masks for the doctor and nurse. These are put on when entering, and removed when leaving the room.

The Nurse. Her hands must be kept free from cracks and cuts. She should frequently use an antiseptic gargle (*e.g.* permanganate of potash) if it is a disease spread by droplet infection.

Terminal Disinfection.

(When the patient is well and free from infection.)

The nurse wears a clean gown.

The Patient. His clothing is removed and he is wrapped in a big towel or gown and taken to the bathroom, where he has a warm bath, to which disinfectant may be added. The hair is washed and a gargle given. He is wrapped in a clean bathgown, taken to another room, and dressed in clean clothes. The nurse then disposes of the contents of the room in the manner described below.

Toys, books, and all articles of little value are burnt.

Linen. This is soaked in disinfectant for twelve hours and sent to the laundry.

Crockery and Other Utensils. These are boiled.

Mattresses, Pillows and Blankets. These are taken for disinfection to the public disinfecting station.

Floors, fixtures and furniture are scrubbed, washed, or polished as is most suitable, and the room is well aired and thoroughly cleaned.

Barrier Nursing

This is carried out in a general ward.

Position. A corner bed is chosen, if possible, and screened, or some other distinguishing sign used. A wide space must be reserved round the bed.

Three tables, shelves or trolleys are in the screened space:

1. For crockery—all marked, or preferably of a special colour or pattern.

2. For toilet utensils—all marked, or of a special pattern.

3. For dressings, if needed, and treatment trays.

One nurse, if possible, attends to the patient. No one else passes the barrier.

Cleaning inside the barrier is done only by this nurse.

Three gowns hang inside. The nurse wears one when inside the barrier. She removes it on coming out, and scrubs her hands and arms.

Linen
Bedpans
Excreta
Food
} Precautions are taken as before.

For special measures of control and modes of transmission of diseases, see Chapter XVI.

HYGIENE OF THE WARD AND
SICK ROOM

Much under this heading will be in the nature of recapitulation and will therefore be summarized briefly.

Hygiene of the Ward

Heating and Ventilation. Central heating with a coal or electric fire for convalescents is the ideal for wards. The temperature should be about 60° F. except in recovery wards where it should be rather warmer. In summer any available blinds should be used to keep out direct sun at midday while the maximum of air inlet is arranged. Exhaust ventilators fitted in windows or walls are excellent; electric fans, too, are useful, especially if placed by an open window. Cross ventilation may sometimes be helpful.

Sluice Rooms, Lavatories, Testing Rooms and Bathrooms. Sluices, lavatory pans, sinks and baths must be kept perfectly clean and disinfected, also shelves, racks, utensils, and specimen cupboards. Specimens should not be left about, but be put in the place provided. Linen and dressing bins must be kept covered, and cleaned and disinfected at the proper times. Floors should be cleaned with suction sweepers and either washed or polished. Leaking pipes or faulty washers should be reported at once.

Cleaning. Damp dusting and polishing are the methods used. "High dusting" is unnecessary in modern wards where there are no ledges or corners. Dust may be responsible for cross-infection. The tubercle bacillus and hæmolytic streptococcus in particular are highly resistant organisms and may be the cause of dust-borne infection. The feet of furniture, screens, etc., need special attention.

Lighting. Diffused light from big centre lights, with local direct (opaque) lights over beds and other places

5*

where required, is perhaps the most useful method. Coloured bulbs may replace white ones at night over beds where observation is needed.

The Ward Kitchen. All tables, shelves, and cupboards must be kept spotlessly clean. The washing sink and draining board require special care. The sink tray should not be left with remains of food in it, and pipes and traps must not be blocked with food or grease. A good detergent should be used for cleaning.

The food bin should contain food refuse only, and the general refuse bin all other rubbish. Both must be emptied and cleaned out daily.

Larders and refrigerators should be cleaned out daily, also bread bins; all receptacles used for milk must be scalded with boiling water after washing. All food should be covered and flies must be killed with some fly-catching device.

Washing-up must be supervised so that really hot water is used and plenty of it. Mops and brushes should be washed in boiling water and put in the sun or air daily.

Gas or electric stoves are washed inside and out, using a detergent. Leaks, whether gas or water, must be repaired at once.

The floor is washed every day, brooms and brushes are washed on the appointed days, and clean drying cloths are provided daily.

There should be no waste of gas, electricity, or water.

The kitchen should always look fresh and clean and tidy.

General Points. Modern wards have as few things as possible about, and, provided there are flowers, this gives a sense of rest and not of bareness.

Ward colourings, though not under control of the nurse, are much studied. Cream walls are nearly always right, dark colours are depressing, green and blue are restful, red is violently irritating, and yellow is displeasing to the sick. Vivid colours and startling patterns should not be chosen for screen covers, curtains, etc. They may become almost intolerable to patients who have to lie and look at them continually.

Patients' lockers should be kept clean inside and tidy outside, and this is usually possible without sweeping all their possessions away.

Ward Atmosphere. This is real but intangible, and affects both the patients and nurses. The nursing staff creates the atmosphere and the patients react to it. The ward sister naturally has most influence, but each nurse has her share of responsibility for it. An atmosphere of happiness and confidence is of great value to the patients. It will exist wherever nurses are devoted to their work and co-operate with each other.

Hygiene of the Sick Room

The Room. If there is a choice, the room should be one into which the sun shines at least during some part of the day, but a noisy position should be avoided. If a room with a balcony is available, it will be a great asset. If it is overloaded with furniture and ornaments, a tactful nurse can usually remove some of these. She can then place the bed where the patient has a view out of the window without directly facing it, and she will probably find a screen very useful.

Heating, Cooling and Ventilation. *In Winter.* The nurse is fortunate if she has a coal fire, in spite of the work and dust made, for ventilation is much easier, the air fresher, and the effect cheerful. If there is a gas or electric fire, a single window, even with the wall ventilators provided, does not keep the air moving across the room sufficiently, as a rule, without the help of an electric fan or of the door at times. The temperature should be about 60° F., and no unpleasant smells from dressings or bedpans, or odours of cooking, should be tolerated. One or two air-wicks will keep the air fresh, and after use of the bedpan the patient should be covered up and windows and doors thrown open for a few minutes.

In Summer. Every effort must be made to keep the patient cool. Blinds and sun blinds will keep out direct sunshine, and green is the best colour to choose. The still, hot air is very trying to the patient, and an electric fan if it is available will give him more relief than anything. If possible it should be placed before an open window, or a dish of ice may be placed in front of it, the mere sight of which will suggest coolness.

The sheets should be drawn or changed, the pillows turned often, and cooling lotions used for sponging. Windows open after dark may cause trouble with mosquitos and moths, but a light wooden frame made the right size and covered with netting can easily be hung on hooks over the open window and removed in the daytime.

Lighting. Strong sunlight should be shaded from the patient's eyes, and at night the table lamp must be adjusted for his comfort.

Cleaning. This should be done with as little discomfort for the patient as possible. A mop for a wooden floor or linoleum, and if possible a vacuum cleaner for the carpets (unless the noise worries the patient), are best. A modern room is easy to keep clean, but one that is over-furnished will need a little tactful clearing.

Flowers should be removed at night so that they may be rearranged in the morning.

Food. Meals should be served as daintily as it is possible to manage. The meal tray should be a studied work of art if the necessaries are available. Spotless china, silver and linen, the colour scheme carried out in the flowers on the tray, and the quantities small and temptingly served, will arouse the patient's interest in his meal. Colouring can be varied with very small expense, and a little trouble is well worth while.

The patient should not know what is coming. Drinks (covered) and fruit may be on the bedside table, but no other food should be left.

The Nurse. Above all, the nurse should be sympathetic and gentle, making her patients feel that her whole concern is for their comfort. She should give an impression of complete reliability and, whatever she may feel, she must never appear anxious. She should move about quietly, and she will do well to consider that the voice has a great power of influence. So also has appearance, and uniform should be correct, spotless and properly worn. Tact, consideration and adaptability are all invaluable, and discord should be kept out of the sick room, where the nurse should aim at securing an atmosphere of peace.

An over-talkative nurse may be very tiring to a really ill patient, and the sick are easily irritated by little things that they would not notice if they were well.

If a nurse really has the good of her patient at heart, she is not likely to be inconsiderate in word or deed, and she will know how to meet the difficulties that must arise at times in the houses where she nurses, without upsetting the patient's relatives or losing her own peace of mind. She bears a great responsibility, since the good name of her own hospital, and the nursing profession as a whole, will be judged by her attitude and behaviour.

CHAPTER X

PARASITES AND HOUSE PESTS

Fig. 39 shows the more important of the parasites and insects that cause and carry disease, and the groups to which they belong. Some of these, printed in italics, are subjects for more advanced study. They are included to make the table more comprehensive.

PARASITES

A parasite is an organism, either vegetable or animal, that lives on or in another creature which is spoken of as its "host", and from which it obtains its nourishment.

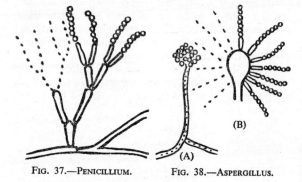

Fig. 37.—Penicillium.   Fig. 38.—Aspergillus.

Vegetable Parasites

Moulds. These are fungi that form spores. There are many different kinds. Figs. 37 and 38 show the structure of two moulds as seen under the microscope.

Moulds on Food. These growths form on bread, meat, fruit, milk, jam, cheese, etc. They consist of tiny threads, each having a cluster of spores, either attached to it, or in little "cases". The cases burst, the spores scatter, and the mould spreads. The effect of mould on food is to decompose it, causing an unpleasant taste and producing acid.

Some moulds are used commercially, as in making Stilton cheese and in medicine. One mould produces penicillin, another streptomycin, another chloromycetin, and others may yet be found to have similar valuable uses.

Ringworm (Tinea). This is an affection of the skin caused by a sporing fungus which penetrates into the hair follicles and destroys the hairs; these break off leaving stumps scattered over ring-shaped scaly patches, which soon become yellow and crusted. There are different types of the fungus, affecting the scalp, body, beard area, nails, and also the skin of animals. The affected hairs are highly infectious, since they are loaded with innumerable spores. Treatment of ringworm of the scalp:

1. *Epilation.* The hair must be made to fall out since it is otherwise impossible to reach the roots in order to kill the fungus. First the hair is cut short all over the scalp, and then made to fall out either by—

   (*a*) X-ray exposures, the doses being carefully measured since an overdose would cause permanent baldness.

   (*b*) Thallium acetate given by mouth, also in carefully measured doses because it is a poisonous drug.

2. *Treatment of the Scalp.* It should be washed every day, and usually either painting with tincture of iodine or application of disinfectant ointment is ordered, since

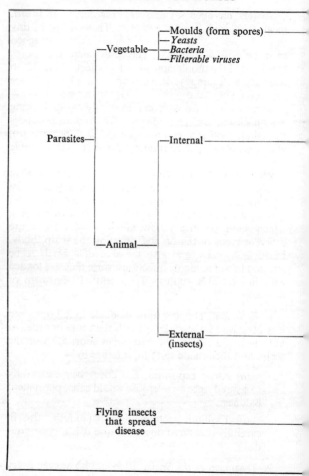

FIG. 39.—IMPORTANT DISEA

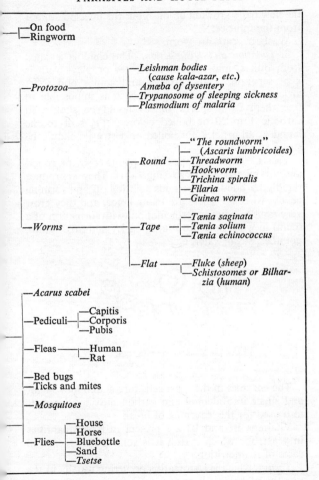

┌─ On food
└─ Ringworm

─ Protozoa ─── Leishman bodies
                 (cause kala-azar, etc.)
               Amœba of dysentery
               Trypanosome of sleeping sickness
               Plasmodium of malaria

─ Worms ─── Round ─── "The roundworm"
                        (Ascaris lumbricoides)
                      Threadworm
                      Hookworm
                      Trichina spiralis
                      Filaria
                      Guinea worm

            Tape ─── Tænia saginata
                     Tænia solium
                     Tænia echinococcus

            Flat ─── Fluke (sheep)
                     Schistosomes or Bilharzia (human)

─ Acarus scabei

─ Pediculi ─── Capitis
              Corporis
              Pubis

─ Fleas ─── Human
            Rat

─ Bed bugs
─ Ticks and mites

─ Mosquitoes

─ Flies ─── House
            Horse
            Bluebottle
            Sand
            Tsetse

CARRYING PARASITES AND INSECTS.

the new hairs growing up push out the infected stumps from the follicles.

Washable caps are worn.

3. *Isolation and Disinfection.* The child is isolated from others, and everything it uses or plays with is kept separate. Hats, brushes and combs and toilet articles should be destroyed since it is impossible to free them from spores; linen should be soaked in carbolic 1 in 20 or boiled before being sent to the laundry; all articles not boiled or destroyed should be steam sterilized.

Yeasts. These are one-celled plants, oval or round and of microscopic size (Fig. 40). They reproduce rapidly by budding, the buds splitting off and forming new yeast cells. There are many kinds, and they grow very rapidly, causing fermentation (with formation of a scum) in wine, beer, fruit juice, barley and other grain, potatoes, sugar water, etc.

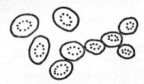

FIG. 40.—YEAST CELLS (SACCHAROMYCES).

The enzymes in the yeast cells turn starch into sugar, and sugar into alcohol and carbon dioxide. Yeast is also used for the leavening of bread.

Vitamins B1 and B2 are present in large quantities in yeast, for which reason it is sometimes ordered in cases of malnutrition.

Thrush, which is a stomatitis occurring usually in the mouths of babies, is caused by a fungus of the yeast type.

Bacteria. Almost all the known bacteria are considered to belong to the vegetable kingdom; the types are discussed in Chapter IX.

Filterable viruses are probably responsible for many of the infectious diseases of which the organisms have not yet been isolated.

Animal Parasites

External Parasites.

Acarus scabiei. Disease caused—scabies.

This is a member of the large group of acari, the other members attacking only animals.

The Acarus is a round, white, shiny, eyeless mite, tiny, but just visible, provided with a sucker, and legs with bristles. The male stays on the skin surface, but the female burrows into the skin, making a little tunnel along the course of which she lays in the space of a week or two about thirty eggs, after which she dies. The eggs hatch out in a few days and the larvæ creep out on to the skin, and soon become adult. After mating, the females again bore tunnels in which to lay their eggs. Intense irritation is caused by the mites crawling about on the skin. The "burrows" can be seen, looking like wavy black lines, and the favourite places are, between the fingers and the toes, the backs of the hands, the front of wrists, the knees, elbows, axillæ and feet; the face is seldom attacked. Children scratch, making sore places, and if these are infected a condition of impetigo may result.

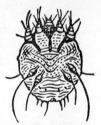

FIG. 41.—ACARUS SCABIEI.

Treatment. A hot bath is given. Then, in a warm room, emulsion of benzyl benzoate is applied over the whole body and limbs, especially between the fingers and toes and round the wrists. This must dry in thoroughly, so the patient waits about 15 to 20 minutes before dressing. For two days the patient must not bath, and after washing the hands a little of the emulsion should be applied. One treatment is a cure. An alternative method is to paint the patient all over with a watery solution of benzyl benzoate after a hot bath,

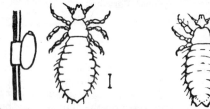

FIG. 42.—PEDICULUS CAPITIS.   FIG. 43.—PEDICULUS CORPORIS.

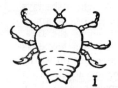

FIG. 44.—PEDICULUS PUBIS.

repeating the painting in 5 minutes, and repeating the bath in 24 hours. The emulsion method is less trouble and less unpleasant.

Lice (pediculi). There are three varieties that attack man.

Pediculus capitis (the head louse). There are two conditions for which head lice are often responsible:

Swollen glands at the back of the neck and ears.

Impetigo due to scratching and infection of the sores.

It is a little, light-greyish insect that lives on the scalp. Its six legs all have claws, with which it hangs on the hairs, and its head has a sucker with which to puncture the skin and suck blood. When not in use, the sucker is retracted within the head. The eggs, called nits, are white and each is in a little case which is stuck to the hair with a cement-like substance secreted by the louse. The eggs are laid close to the scalp, but as the hair grows they are seen lower down, the nape of the neck and behind the ears being favourite places. The female lays sixty or more eggs in a month, which hatch in a week, and the lice are full-grown in ten to twenty-one days.

The exudate caused by their bites forms crusts and mats the hair.

They leave the heads of patients with very high temperatures, and also the dying.

Treatment. 1. Suleo, an emulsion of D.D.T. in liquid paraffin is applied to the hair and scalp, followed by washing and fine combing after some hours. The treatment is continued for a week since D.D.T. kills the lice as they hatch out from the nits.

2. Lethane oil is sometimes applied, followed by a shampoo in three or more days. This is not considered a satisfactory treatment.

3. The older treatment of a sassafras compress is still sometimes used.

Pediculus corporis (the body louse). Diseases carried or caused:

> Typhus fever.
> Trench fever.
> Septic dermatitis (caused by scratching).
> Relapsing fever.

The insect is much like the head louse, but a little larger. It bites the body and sucks blood causing intense irritation. It is found in the clothes, especially down the seams. The female lays the eggs on the clothing in seams or folds, about thirty a week during a life of four to five weeks. They are white and very tiny, and they hatch out in seven to ten days. The lice become mature in two weeks.

Treatment. Delousing is carried out by blowing D.D.T. powder (5 per cent. D.D.T. in an inert powder) under the clothing and on the skin, using a hand blower. This kills the lice but not the nits. The infected person is then undressed, and both skin and clothing are again treated.

D.D.T. powder is used in the same way for prevention.

Pediculus pubis (the pubic louse). The same diseases are carried.

In shape it is flatter, and its six legs have strong claws, hence it is sometimes called the "crab louse". It lives in the pubic hair, or the axillary hair, or occasionally in the eyebrows.

Each female lays about twelve eggs which hatch in a week.

Treatment. As for body lice.

Fleas—Pulex irritans (the human flea).

There are four stages in the life of the flea:

3-10 Days: Egg.	About 2 Weeks: Larva.	About 2 Weeks: Pupa.	Adult.
This is large and white, laid in bedding, dust and rubbish, cracks in floor and furniture.	Emerges from the eggs; has neither eyes nor legs. Feeds on any organic matter —e.g., dead flies, etc. Spins a cocoon inside which it changes into a pupa.	The cocoon remains in the dust in some crack. Inside it the pupa is changing into a flea, and it may live on in the cocoon for as long as four months.	The flea emerges from the cocoon. Time taken from egg to adult, about five or six weeks, but can be as short as ten days.

The adult flea has a horny brown skin, hooked feet, and very large strong back legs for jumping. It lives on the blood that it sucks and if well fed can live many months, but without food it dies in a few days.

The irritation caused by their bites induces scratching,

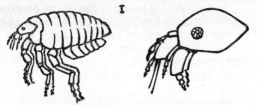

FIG. 45.—PULEX IRRITANS (the Human Flea).

and septic infection may enter through the bites or scratches.

To get rid of fleas:

1. All dust, dirt and old bedding, clothing and carpets should be cleared away.

2. The room and all furniture should be scrubbed with soap and water, and sun and air allowed to enter.

3. D.D.T. powder is blown into all cracks round the floor and walls, and into the furniture and bedding.

Rat flea (Xenopsylla cheopis) is the carrier of plague. Plague is a disease that attacks rats, which die in thousands when there is an epidemic among them. Fleas on the infected rats suck the blood of their hosts and take in with it thousands of plague bacilli. The rat dies, and its fleas seeking a new host will go to humans if any are near. When they bite, they regurgitate the living plague bacilli into the man.

Prevention of Plague in Western Countries.

1. All ships unloading cargo, especially grain, are searched for dead rats, and any found are examined by the city bacteriologist for plague bacilli.

2. Ships may be either—

(*a*) *Infected*, if there is a case of plague on board, or if a case has developed more than six days after embarkation, or if plague-infected rats have been found.

(*b*) *Suspected*, if a case of plague has developed within six days of embarkation, or if there has been a high and unexplained mortality among rats.

In both cases the ship is isolated, and if *infected* the procedure is:

(1) The ship is inspected and all on board examined.

(2) The sick are disembarked and isolated.

(3) Contacts are either isolated or placed under surveillance.

(4) Bedding, etc., is disinfected.

(5) Infected parts of the ship are disinfected.

(6) The ship, if necessary, is "deratized". This is done by hydrocyanic acid gas, the parts under treatment being carefully sealed.

For *suspected* ships, numbers (1), (4), (5), and (6) apply.

3. Ships calling at ports where there are cases of plague have "rat guards" (shaped like lamp shades, with the small end fitting the rope and wide end facing the quay) on their mooring-ropes, so that rats cannot run up to the ship.

4. At home ports the Port Health Officers who board the ship receive reports of, and deal with, any cases of infection.

5. Grain stores and warehouses should be built with concrete floors and concrete footings to the walls.

6. Warehouses, quays and sheds are constantly searched for dead rats, and rat-killing measures are in constant use. All rats are examined for plague bacilli,

and the number of *rat fleas* capable of carrying plague are estimated. This is called the *cheopis index*, and whenever it rises above normal for the port, anti-rat measures are intensified.

Bugs. Bed Bugs (Cimex lectularius). It is not proved that bugs carry disease in this country, but they cause irritation and annoyance and loss of sleep. In tropical countries they may carry leishmaniasis, typhus and relapsing fever, and are known experimentally to be capable of carrying plague. They live in cracks in walls, floor, woodwork, furniture, and especially beds, and at night they come out, bite the occupants of the beds and suck blood, the bite causing great irritation. The eggs are laid in some crack, two, three or more at a time (200 or so in all). They hatch in a week, and grow to adults in six weeks if food is plentiful, or some months if it is scarce. The adult is flat, oval and brownish-red, and produces an oily secretion which causes an unpleasant musty smell. They can live eight to nine months without food, becoming as thin as paper. They travel in wall spaces from room to room and are extremely difficult to eradicate.

Methods of extermination are:

1. Removal of broken woodwork.

2. Fumigation with sulphur or hydrocyanic gas.

3. D.D.T. powder blown into cracks, and round woodwork.

4. Paraffin oil squirted into cracks with an oilcan (done after dark when bugs come out, but with due precaution against fire).

5. Repeated scrubbing with soap and water, and airing of rooms.

6. Untiring repetition of these measures.

7. Destruction of bug-infested property.

8. Care that infected furniture does not carry them to a fresh house. When removing families from slum areas to new houses, it is sometimes the practice to fumigate the family possessions in the removal van by leaving the van for a few hours filled with hydrocyanic acid gas.

Black beetles are said to eat bed bugs.

Ticks and Mites. This is a large class of insects, including varying types, found in all countries of the world. All kinds bite and suck the blood of humans or animals.

The harvest bug is a well-known type.

Internal Parasites.

Worms—Roundworms (Nematodes). The following are the chief varieties that are parasitic in man:

The Common Roundworm (Ascaris lumbricoides). *Appearance.* Pale greyish-white or pinkish in colour

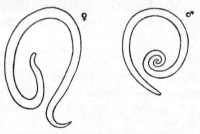

FIG. 46.—THE COMMON ROUNDWORM.

like an earthworm, 6–16 inches long, the female being longer than the male.

Life. The eggs are taken in with food or water which has been contaminated with them. The capsule is dissolved in the stomach, and the larvæ develop in the intestines and then pass through the intestinal wall, and travelling in lymph and blood they reach the lungs. Here they undergo further changes, after which they pass up the trachea, into the pharynx, down the œsophagus to the stomach and back to the intestines. Here they live, and the female lays many yellow oval eggs, thick coated, with a rough surface, which are passed in the stools and may contaminate water or uncooked salad foods. Sometimes the worm wanders up the bile duct or pancreatic duct, or into the œsophagus and is vomited.

Prevention. In those hot countries where the worm is commonly found unboiled water and uncooked vegetables and salads should never be taken.

Threadworm (Oxyuris vermicularis). *Appearance.* The worms appear in the stool like little white threads with pointed head and tail. The male, which is too small to be seen easily, has its tail incurved.

Life. The eggs are taken into the child's mouth from its infected fingers or food that it has handled. In the stomach the capsules dissolve, and the embryos pass down to the intestine, where they live. The fertilized females are present in large numbers in the cæcum and colon and are passed with their ova in the stools.

At night the females migrate to the anus and cause intense irritation. The child scratches, gets both eggs and worms on the fingers and round the nails, and if he has the habit of thumb-sucking he swallows these and reinfects his alimentary canal.

Symptoms. Intense irritation round the anus at night, sleeplessness, eczema from scratching, enuresis, convulsions, disorders of appetite.

Prevention. This is achieved by keeping the nails short and clean, seeing that the child wears gloves at night, frequent changing of bed linen, underclothes, pyjamas and towels. He should sleep alone, and

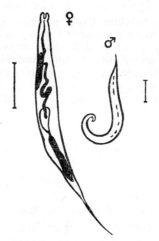

FIG. 47.—THE THREADWORM.

mercurial ointment may be applied round the anus at night to allay irritation.

Hookworm (Ankylostoma duodenale). *Appearance.* The worm is about half an inch long, and the mouth contains hooked spines with which it attaches itself to the wall of the duodenum.

Life. The eggs are laid in the intestine and pass out in the fæces. If they are deposited in warm damp soil, as in mines or in tropical countries, the eggs hatch in a few days, and the larvæ after several months are fully developed. They remain in wet earth or on grass, and pierce bare skin, travelling through the blood stream to the duodenum where they fasten their hooks into the wall and suck the blood of their hosts.

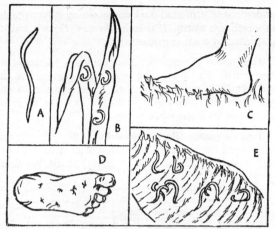

FIG. 48—THE HOOKWORM.

Ova of the worm are passed in the fæces and in warm damp earth they develop into larvæ which pierce the skin and travel in lymph and blood circulations to the intestines.

(A) Worm, natural size; (B) Worm on grass; (C) Foot among infected grass; (D) Larvæ pierce and enter the skin; (E) Worms attached to the lining of the intestines.

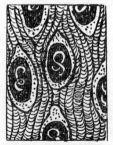

FIG. 49—"MEASLY" PORK.

Trichina spiralis. Man is infected by this worm through the eating of infected pork which has been undercooked. Infected pork contains tiny cysts in each of which is a worm. It is called "measly" pork and is discarded by meat inspectors.

Tapeworms (Cestodes). Two common varieties of tapeworms, *Tænia saginata* and *Tænia solium*, live in the human intestines, and their cystic stage is in an animal, while *Tænia echinococcus* has its worm stage in a dog and its cystic stage in man.

Tænia saginata (Beef tapeworm). *Life.* The worm lives in the human intestines and may grow to 20 or 24 feet in length. Its head, which is very small, has four

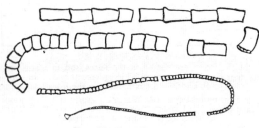

FIG. 50—BEEF TAPEWORM.

suckers with which it attaches itself to the wall of the intestine. The rest of the worm consists of thin whitish rectangular segments, which are small near the head and gradually increase in size. The larger segments are full of ova (the worm is a hermaphrodite, each segment containing male and female reproductive organs). The segments break off and are passed in the stools; and should such stools be passed where a stream or grass can be infected, a bullock may swallow the ova, which then develop into embryos and pass from the stomach of the animal to its muscles, where each embryo becomes encysted. When the animal is killed for food, the cysts should be discovered during inspection; otherwise, should the beef be undercooked, the cysts will develop in the intestines of the persons who eat it, and produce new tapeworms.

Symptoms. Usually the infected person sees segments in a stool. There may be indigestion, colic, and either

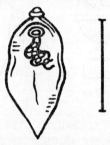

FIG. 51.—HEAD OF BEEF TAPEWORM.

anorexia or voracious or perverted appetite. Anæmia and nerve symptoms sometimes occur.

If, after treatment for expulsion of the worm, the head is left behind, the worm will grow again.

Prevention. This is by careful meat inspection, and by avoiding undercooked meat.

Tænia solium (Pork tapeworm). This is a smaller worm, 6–12 feet long, sometimes called the "armed tapeworm" because its head has a ring of hooks as well as four suckers, with which to attach itself to the wall of the intestines. The patient often has several worms. The cyst stage is in the pig, and infection is from eating "measly pork" insufficiently cooked, generally in sausages.

Another type of tapeworm has its cystic stage in freshwater fish and is only killed by sufficient cooking.

THE PORK TAPEWORM

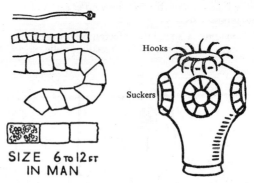

SIZE 6 to 12 FT
IN MAN

FIG. 52.—HEAD AND SEGMENTS.   FIG. 53.—HEAD.

FIG. 54.—EGG OF PORK TAPEWORM.   FIG. 55.—CYSTICERCUS.

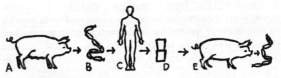

FIG. 56.—INFECTION STAGES OF PORK TAPEWORM.

(A) Infected pig; (B) Uncooked sausages; (C) Infected man;
(D) Broken-off segments; (E) Pig infected.

In all types salting and pickling of meat and fish fail to kill the cyst.

Tænia echinococcus.   This worm lives in the intestines of dogs, and has its cyst stage in man. The worm is only about half an inch long, and has three or four segments, and a head provided with suckers and hooks. The end segment contains eggs, which are passed in the

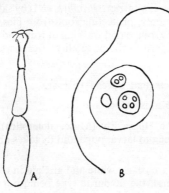

FIG. 57.
TÆNIA ECHINOCOCCUS (the Dog Tapeworm).
(A) The worm; (B) Hydatid cyst containing "daughter" cysts in the human liver.

fæces. These may contaminate water, or grass, or even food which has been touched after handling an infected dog. In this way man, cattle or sheep may swallow ova from which the embryo escape and travel in the blood to the liver where they form a "hydatid cyst". This cyst may grow very large, and in it there develop "daughter and grand-daughter cysts". The cysts may also occur in the lungs, kidneys or brain.

This condition is common in Iceland, where dogs are much in the house, and in Australia and other sheep-farming countries.

6

Prevention is by avoiding contaminating the hands with the fæces of dogs.

Amœba of Dysentery. These amœbæ attack the colon, causing severe ulceration, and are passed in the fæces. As the disease becomes chronic the amœbæ are encysted, and the cysts in the stools may reach food either by contaminated water or by flies, or by the hands of a person who is a carrier. *Prophylaxis* is by safeguarding the water supply, protecting food from flies, care with regard to the source and washing of fruit and salad, and also with regard to the possibility of carriers.

Flying Insects that Spread Disease.

These are mosquitoes and flies.

Flies—The House Fly (Musca domestica). The life cycle from egg to larva, pupa and fly takes about ten or twelve days.

The eggs are pearly white and are laid in moist, warm organic refuse, the favourite type being horse manure, but human fæces, decaying vegetable matter or any fermenting refuse is used by the fly. About 100 eggs are laid at a time and four or five batches in a season.

The larvæ hatch out in about twenty-four hours and in four or five days are fully grown. Then, in some crack or refuse heap, they change into *pupæ*. In a few days more the pupa becomes an *adult fly*. The body and legs of the fly are hairy, and on them bacteria are carried from one place to another. The feet have both claws and sticky pads (so that it can cling to surfaces upside down) and to these also germs adhere. The head is mobile with compound eyes. For feeding it has a proboscis, so, unable to eat solid food, it must first dissolve its meal. This it does with saliva. Settling for instance on sugar, it regurgitates saliva on to it, and then sucks it up through its proboscis. It often vomits this again on the food or elsewhere and also defæcates

THE HOUSE FLY

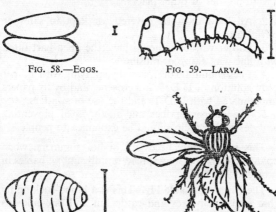

FIG. 58.—EGGS. FIG. 59.—LARVA.

FIG. 60.—PUPA. FIG. 61.—ADULT FLY.

leaving "fly-spots". Bacteria remain alive in a fly's intestines and are excreted during these proceedings, so that its feeding habits may easily spread disease. Diseases carried by flies are enteric fever, dysentery, epidemic diarrhœa, cholera, and tropical ophthalmia.

Prevention of Flies. 1. Breeding places must not be allowed to exist; therefore—

    (*a*) Collections of dirt and refuse must be removed.

    (*b*) Refuse bins must be kept covered, and emptied and cleaned out frequently.

    (*c*) Horse manure should not be left about.

(*d*) Privies, if they must be retained, should be cleaned out regularly, and the stools always covered with earth or ashes.

(*e*) Dumps of vegetable refuse should not remain in pigsties or other places.

2. All food must be covered, or kept in safes or refrigerators.

3. Larder windows should have the open part fitted with fine wire gauze or muslin.

4. Flies should be destroyed by spraying with a 5 per cent. solution of D.D.T. in kerosene, and by fly papers impregnated with D.D.T. and the use of swatters.

5. The danger of flies and methods of preventing and destroying them should be explained to people.

This is especially necessary in hot summers, when epidemic diarrhœa may spread rapidly among babies in crowded areas.

The Horse or Stable Fly. This is a blood-sucking fly that feeds on horses and cattle but will bite humans quite readily. It may spread anthrax among cattle.

Bluebottle and Greenbottle Flies. These are larger than house flies, and they breed in meat or any decaying animal matter, on which the larvæ feed. They spread bacteria in the same way as do house flies.

Mosquitoes carry the parasite of *malaria* and the virus of *yellow fever* and *dengue fever*.

Malaria. The mosquito that carries the parasite of malaria is the female of the Anopheles variety which, on alighting, rests on its two front pairs of legs, raising its back pair in the air. The *eggs* are laid on the surface of stagnant water in ponds, garden tanks, marshes, or any receptacle. The *larvæ* hatch out and float on the surface of the water, since they must have air to breathe. They live on minute water plants and organisms. The *pupa* stage is short, and finally the *mosquito* emerges. The

THE ANOPHELES MOSQUITO

In figures 63 and 64 note the air intake tubes.

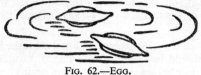

Fig. 62.—Egg.

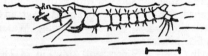

Fig. 63.—Larva.

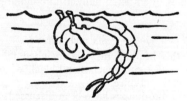

Fig. 64. Pupa.

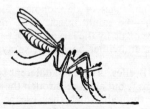

Fig. 65.—Anopheles.

cycle, in the tropics, may be completed in ten days.
The male lives entirely on vegetation, but the female
bites any creature and sucks blood through a proboscis,
while at the same time injecting fluid into the bite from
its salivary glands. Should the mosquito have bitten
previously someone suffering from malaria, it will inject
the parasite into the blood of any persons it may bite
subsequently.

Prophylaxis. In mosquito-infested areas the breeding
places should be destroyed; no stagnant water should
remain near houses; even broken jars or tins containing
water will become breeding grounds. Large areas of
water are drained or sprayed with kerosene and D.D.T.
so that the larvæ die for want of air. Paris green (copper
aceto-arsenite) is also used for spraying. Water weeds
should first be cleared.

Spraying with a 5 per cent. solution of D.D.T. is
valuable in houses.

Quinine is often taken daily in infested areas.

House Pests and Vermin

Under this heading may be included flies, moths,
furniture beetles, cockroaches and blackbeetles and the
rodents—rats and mice.

Flies and mosquitoes have been discussed.

Moths. The house moth will destroy any organic
material. The stages of development are: egg, larva,
pupa, moth—the adult insect. The moth holes in
materials are made by the larvæ. D.D.T. destroys them
at all stages, and either powder or spray may be used.

Furniture Beetles. There are different species of these
"woodworms", but all bore through the wood, making
flight holes through which they escape, infesting adjacent wood. One species—the death watch beetle—

does great damage in oak beams of ancient buildings causing them to rot away. All types are destroyed by squirting special "timber fluids" into the tunnels and painting it over the surrounding wood.

Cockroaches and Blackbeetles. These pests are found in warm places, *e.g.* under cookers, behind hot water tanks and hot pipes. The eggs are deposited in cracks, especially in wooden fittings. There is a special emulsion of D.D.T. which may be painted on the floor around the fixtures, and injected into the cracks, but first, all foodstuffs must be removed and the windows must be opened, and kept open until the odour of the insecticide has disappeared. D.D.T. is a contact poison so it must be applied where the insects will run over it. In extreme cases a Disinfestation Service may be called upon and it may be necessary to open up floors, laying bare the hot pipes for more thorough treatment.

Rodents. Rats and mice are a serious menace. They thrive in dirty surroundings and slum conditions. Bad housing, garbage and refuse heaps, and faulty sewage disposal provide suitable breeding conditions for them. They also infest grain stores, barns and farm premises, and rats are always present in the holds of ships. (See page 151). Mice are liable to appear anywhere where food remains and crumbs are left about. Methods for protection against, and ridding premises of these vermin include:

1. No food scraps should be left about; empty cake and biscuit tins should be kept free from crumbs; no food, bread bins, etc., should be left uncovered.

2. Holes through walls and floors should be efficiently sealed.

3. The occasional odd mouse may be destroyed by various poison baits, provided there are no domestic animals about.

4. In the event of persistent infestation, and always in the case of rat infestation, a Rodent Officer should be called in, or a Disinfestation Service employed. These experts will discover the source of the infestation and seal the runways, as well as destroying the pests. If necessary a Public Health Inspector may investigate the adjacent buildings and order suitable treatment.

CHAPTER XI

FOOD AND FOOD VALUES

THE body is built, kept in repair and enabled to work by means of the food that is taken into it.

All foods are broken down by chemical processes into simple substances which are carried round in solution in blood and lymph and absorbed by the tissue cells which pick out all they need for their life and work.

The food substances are utilized for the following purposes:

1. To build up and keep in repair the cell substance.

2. To combine with oxygen in producing energy for the varied work of the cells, and also heat.

3. To provide the mineral substances that the cells require.

4. To regulate the body processes and provide protection from various unhealthy conditions.

5. To keep right the water balance of the body.

A good diet must contain all that is needed by the body cells for their life and work, and is therefore made up of the following types of food.

Make-up of a good diet.
—**Protein**—for building and repairing cells.
—**Carbohydrate**—for burning, to do cell work and make heat, and for storage fuel.
—**Fat**—for reserve fuel.
—**Mineral Salts**—for cell activities.
—**Protective Substances**—vitamins, to assist the cells with their chemical processes, and so protect the body against disease.
—**Water**—to maintain water balance.
—**Roughage**—to stimulate bowel excretion.

6*

Proteins are composed of carbon, hydrogen, oxygen, *nitrogen,* sulphur and phosphorus.

No other food contains nitrogen.

Their use is to repair and to build up the body tissues.

When digested they are broken down into amino acids which build up cell protoplasm. Excess amino acids are broken down in the liver, the carbon, hydrogen and oxygen being re-synthesized to produce carbohydrate. Spare protein is therefore a supplementary energy food.

Proteins are present in many foods and vary in value to the body, according to the amino acids they contain.

Examples of Proteins:

1st Class Proteins contain *all* the amino acids needed by the body, and in right proportions. All are animal proteins.	lean meat. fish. eggs—3 proteins: albumin—egg white. vitellin, globulin } in egg yolk. milk—2 proteins: caseinogen. lactalbumin. cheese—caseinogen.
2nd Class Proteins contain *all* the amino acids needed by the body, but not in the right proportions, so that large quantities must be taken in a vegetarian diet.	wheat, oats, maize, barley, rice, bread and oatmeal. peas, beans, and nuts. macaroni and spaghetti.

Examples of Proteins—cont.:

Incomplete Protein
Essential amino
acids are missing. ⎱ gelatin.
Useful as a "pro-
tein-sparer".

Extractives from meat, such as Bovril, Oxo, beef tea, etc., are not proteins. Their chief value is as gastric stimulants.

Carbohydrates. These include starches and sugars: they are composed of carbon, hydrogen and oxygen, and are the energy foods. Starch is eaten in the form of potatoes, wheat (bread and all foods made with flour), oatmeal, rice, tapioca, peas, beans, lentils and barley. Sugars are obtained from sugar cane and beet-root, and are present in fruit, milk and honey. Sugar is formed in the green parts of plants, chiefly in the leaves.

The plant by sucking up water through its roots and breathing in carbon dioxide through its leaves obtains the carbon, hydrogen and oxygen needed, and these are combined to form sugar by means of the green substance chlorophyll in the leaves and the radiant energy of sunlight. Excess oxygen is returned to the air. The process is called "photosynthesis". The sugars in milk and honey are passed to the consumer through the cow and the bee, but they also have been obtained from plants.

Plants can convert excess sugar into starch and store it (*e.g.* potatoes), or into cellulose which forms the fibrous and woody parts of stalks, leaves and fruit.

Carbohydrate food eaten in excess of the body's needs is converted into fat.

The following table shows foods containing a large proportion of carbohydrate:

Starch.	Sugars.	Sugar that needs no digesting.

Bread
Potatoes
Cereals:
  Oatmeal
  Rice
  Pearl Barley
  Shredded wheat, etc.
Flour and cornflour
Tapioca
Peas, beans and lentils
	Sucrose (cane and beet sugar)
	
	Lactose, or milk sugar
	
	Maltose, produced by digestion of starch
		Glucose
		Honey
		Fruit sugar (when separated from the cellular material)

Fats. These are composed of carbon, hydrogen and oxygen. They are used in order to conserve body heat and also as fuel food. When oxidized, they produce more heat than sugar, as they contain more carbon; but they require some sugar for complete combustion, otherwise *ketones* (acids) are produced, which are harmful. Fat is stored as drops of oil in fat cells.

Animal fat is more valuable in diet than vegetable fat, because it contains vitamins A and D.

Some fat foods are:

Animal Fats	**Vegetable Fats**
Butter	Olive Oil
Cream	Nuts
Meat fat—bacon	Chocolate
Egg—in the yolk	Margarine
Cheese	
Fat fish	

Salts are of two kinds:

(*a*) *Organic*, in fruit, vegetables and milk. Acetic, citric, oxalic and other acids in these foods do not cause acidity (with the exception of those in plums). They form carbonates, which are alkaline salts or base, and maintain the reaction of the blood in a state of faint alkalinity.

(*b*) *Mineral Salts.* These are salts of lime, sodium, potassium, magnesium, sulphur, iron, etc., in various combinations.

They have many uses in the body and are of vital importance. They are necessary for:

(1) Building of tissue cells—*e.g.* bone, nerve, etc.

(2) Keeping body fluids at the right reaction—*e.g.* blood, gastric juice.

(3) Contraction of muscle and functioning of nerves.

(4) Supplying red blood cells with hæmoglobin to combine with oxygen.

(5) Maintaining correct osmotic pressure of body fluids.

(6) Formation of gland secretions.

(7) Clotting of blood.

Sources and Uses of Minerals

Sodium. This, in table salt (sodium chloride) and in all foods is essential for life. It is needed by every cell in the body and by all body fluids which contain 0·9 per cent. of salt. The salt balance is adjusted by the passing out of excess salt in the urine. Salt is also lost in sweat, therefore extra salt must be taken in hot climates, by miners, stokers and others who work in great heat, and by anyone after strenuous exercise.

Calcium. This combines with phosphorus to produce calcium phosphate which is needed for: (*a*) the development and growth of bones and teeth; (*b*) the contraction of muscles; (*c*) the clotting of blood. Children and expectant mothers especially need a good supply. The best sources are: dried skim milk and cheese. After these come sardines, milk and milk products, watercress, vegetables and eggs.

Phosphorus. This is needed: (*a*) to combine with calcium for the formation of bones and teeth; (*b*) to keep constant the composition of body fluids; (*c*) by every cell in the body (particularly nerve and gland cells).

The best sources are: cheese, oatmeal, liver, kidney and egg and, after these, bread and milk.

Potassium. This is needed particularly in muscle and red blood cells. It is present in most foods, especially kippers, cod, meat, milk and egg.

Magnesium. This is needed for the composition of bones and teeth. It is present in most foods.

Fluorine. This, in small amounts, is present in drinking water and improves the hardness of teeth. It is found also in bones.

Iron. This is needed for the formation of hæmoglobin in red blood cells, and is therefore necessary for carrying oxygen to the cells. Small amounts only are needed because it is used over again when the red blood cells are broken down. Liver, kidney, beef and egg yolk are the best sources, then follow raisins and watercress.

Copper. A very little of this is required for use with iron in red blood cells. All foods contain very small amounts.

Sulphur. This is needed for cell building. Eggs and vegetables are the best sources of supply.

Iodine. This is found in sea foods and water. Very little is needed, but it is very important for body metabolism. It is used by the thyroid gland in its hormone thyroxin.

Roughage. This is chiefly cellulose, in fruit and vegetables and in brown bread. It is not absorbed, but makes bulk in the intestines, and stimulates peristalsis, so preventing constipation.

Water. This is of utmost importance to the body, and the water balance is most carefully adjusted.

It is two-thirds, or over 60 per cent. of the body weight. It is taken in as fluids and in all foods.

It is needed in and around all cells; for secretions; for oxidation and all chemical changes; for the work of enzymes, to wash out toxins and all waste products; and to regulate body temperature.

VITAMINS

Vitamins are present in various foods, are substances that neither build cells nor produce energy, but are essential in various ways for cell chemistry and are absolutely necessary for good health. Very small quantities are sufficient, but if these are absent from the daily diet serious ill health and diseases result. (These are "deficiency diseases".) It is probable that a great deal of minor ill health is caused by small deficiencies of the various vitamins in the daily diet.

Some vitamins are present in plant life and some are elaborated in the body and are present in animal food, such as milk and liver oils. In many cases the animals have fed on grass and herbage (or, in the case of fish, on smaller fish which live on the green algæ of the sea) and the vitamins formed in them are derived from substances in the vegetation.

Vitamins A, D, E, K are soluble in oils and are therefore "fat-soluble", while vitamins C and the B group are "water-soluble".

Some are less stable than others, and are destroyed by heat and by alkaline reaction, and therefore by cooking and the addition of soda. Cold does not affect them, so that they are preserved in cold storage.

Although their chemical composition is very complex, most of them can now be produced synthetically and, as research proceeds, others will probably be isolated.

VITAMIN A

Sources

Vitamin A is soluble in fats.

It is not destroyed when food is cooked or frozen.

Fish liver oils are the most concentrated source of vitamin A.

Milk, butter, cheese, and eggs contain more vitamin A in the summer when animals are pasture fed.

Vitamin A in these animal foods is called *pre-formed* vitamin A. It is the actual chemical vitamin A itself.

Animal Foods
Whole milk
Egg yolk
Butter
Cheese
Liver
Cod-liver oil
Halibut-liver oil

Vitamin A in carrots is due to an orange pigment—*carotene*.

Carotene is also the source of the vitamin in green vegetables, and the darker the leaves the greater is the vitamin content.

Carotene when absorbed into the body is converted into vitamin A.

Animal foods are the best source since they contain pre-formed vitamin A which needs no converting.

Vegetable Foods
Carrots
Spinach
Watercress
Dried apricots
Dried prunes
Tomato
Cabbage
Green peas

Uses of vitamin A

(1) It is necessary for growth in children.

(2) It is protecting to the skin and lining membranes, particularly of the respiratory and digestive tracts, and the cornea of the eye. If deficient the cells become dry and horny and cannot resist infection.

(3) It is needed by the rod cells in the retina for their function of vision in the dark.

Results of Deficiency
(1) Poor growth.
(2) Catarrh and bronchopneumonia.
(3) Affections of the cornea.
(4) Inability to see quickly in a dim light.

VITAMIN D

Vitamin D is soluble in fats.
It is not destroyed when food is cooked or frozen.

Dairy produce contains more vitamin D in the summer when cows are pasture fed.
This vitamin is called *vitamin D₃*.

Ultra-violet rays, whether from sunlight or ultra-violet ray lamps, acting on ergosterol in the sebum on the skin cause vitamin D to be formed and absorbed into the blood.

If certain foods are exposed to ultra-violet light vitamin D is formed in them.
Margarine is treated in this way. This is known as *vitamin D₂*.

Vitamin D_2 (calciferol) and vitamin D_3 can be manufactured.

Uses of vitamin D
It is needed for the calcification of bone and teeth. Calcium and phosphorus are present in many foods

Sources

Animal Fats
Cod- and halibut-liver oil
Sardines
Herrings
Tinned salmon
Egg
Butter
Cheese
Milk

Another source of vitamin D:
Ultra-violet rays in sunlight

(see p. 173) and combine to form calcium phosphate in the blood which is needed to make bones and teeth hard, but in the absence of vitamin D the process cannot take place.

Results of Deficiency

(1) Expectant mothers are unable to provide for the developing bones of the foetus which begin to ossify from the third month.

(2) In infants and children rickets results.

(3) In expectant mothers osteo-malacia (a disease resembling rickets) may develop.

THE VITAMIN B GROUP

The vitamins in this group at present identified number at least eleven different substances which are often found in the same foods.
All are soluble in water.

Vitamin B₁ and Aneurine

The action is very complex, and is concerned with the oxidation of sugar in the body cells with production of energy.
It is needed especially for nutrition of nerve cells.

Results of Deficiency

(1) Growth of children is slowed down.

Sources

In the following order:
Yeast
Peanuts
Bacon
Oatmeal
Green peas
Wholemeal bread
Mutton and beef
Potato
Cabbage
Milk

(2) Neuritis develops.

(3) Beri-beri occurs in extreme deficiency with emaciation and paralysis or œdema and heart failure. The disease is common in those parts of the East where the natives live on rice from which the germ and husk have been removed.

Also:
Marmite
Bemax

Vitamin B_2—Riboflavine

Its function, like that of vitamin B_1, is to assist in the oxidation of sugar in the body.

Results of Deficiency

(1) Growth of children is slowed down.

(2) The tongue becomes sore, and cracks occur at the corners of the mouth.

Sources

In the following order:

Yeast, liver, Marmite, cheese, egg, beef, milk, wholemeal bread, bread, potato, beer

Nicotinic Acid

The function of this vitamin is also to assist in the processes by which the body obtains energy from carbohydrate.

Results of Deficiency

(1) Growth of children is slowed down.

(2) The skin becomes rough and red in exposed parts—the face, neck and hands.

(3) The tongue is red and sore.

(4) Pellagra develops with dyspepsia, diarrhoea, and mental symptoms such as confusion dementia.

Sources

In the following order:

Marmite
Yeast
Liver, kidney
Beef, bacon
Wholemeal bread
Peanuts
Cod
Beer
Potato

Pyrodoxin—Vitamin B$_6$

Its function is concerned with growth and with the nutrition of the skin.

Sources

Yeast, liver, cereals, peas and beans

Folic Acid

This vitamin is useful in the cure of some forms of anæmia.

Liver, green vegetables

Vitamin B$_{12}$

This vitamin is needed for the manufacture of red blood cells.

It is also obtained as a by-product of streptomycin, and is given in cases of pernicious (Addison's) anæmia.

Liver

VITAMIN C
Ascorbic Acid

Vitamin C is soluble in water.

It is present in the cells of fruit and vegetables together with an enzyme which destroys the vitamin whenever the plant cells are damaged by cooking or grating.

Vitamin C is lost therefore through:

(a) Heat, especially long slow cooking.

(b) Grating, due to release of the enzyme which destroys the vitamin.

(c) Long storage of fruit and vegetables.

Uses of Vitamin C

(1) It helps with the process of oxidation in the tissue cells.

Sources

Uncooked foods

Blackcurrants
Oranges
Lemons
Grapefruit
Sprouts
Cabbage
Watercress
Potatoes
Lettuce
Onions, carrots
Apples, plums, pears
Rose-hip syrup (has a high content).
Cows' milk (contains a small amount).

(2) It is needed for formation of the substance that holds tissue cells together.

(3) It assists the healing of wounds.

Sprouted grass (contains the vitamin but dry cereals do not).

Deficiency

(1) Growth of children is slowed down.

(2) The gums and mouth become sore and are easily infected.

(3) The healing of wounds and fractures is slow.

(4) Scurvy develops in severe cases, with hæmorrhages under the skin and under the periosteum of long bones, causing the child to scream if touched. The gums and other mucous membranes are inflamed and bleed, and the child is apathetic.

A breast-fed baby will receive enough vitamin C if the mother's diet is good, but orange juice is always given so as to ensure a sufficient amount.

VITAMIN E

This is a fat-soluble vitamin. It is not destroyed by cooking.

Deficiency in the diet may be a contributory cause of abortion in some cases, and vitamin E preparations may therefore be useful in preventing repeated abortions.

Sources

Plant oils, *e.g.* **wheat-germ and olive oil.**
Egg yolk
Lettuce and other green leaves.
Peas and beans.
Milk.

VITAMIN K	Sources
The liver needs vitamin K for the formation of prothrombin which is present in the blood for clotting. If it is deficient, the prothrombin index is low, and the blood clots slowly. If hæmorrhage occurs it may be severe.	Green leaves, spinach, cabbage, etc. Carrots Tomatoes Soya bean Liver

DIET DEFICIENCY DISEASES

These are given under the headings of the various vitamins.

To them may be added:

Iron deficiency—certain forms of anæmia.

Iodine deficiency—non-toxic goitre.

Poor diet generally—children are thin, under-developed and dull, with little or no resistance to disease—in fact, a condition of marasmus.

METABOLISM AND DIET REQUIREMENTS

The chemical changes that take place in the body cells are very complex, and the sum total of all these processes is called **Metabolism.** This includes the breaking down or digestion of foods into simple substances, re-synthesis into other substances, and their use in the cells, including the burning of fuel foods, chiefly sugar, with oxygen; the formation of waste products and their elimination from the body.

Calorie Values. All cell activities involve the burning of sugar with oxygen with the production of energy and heat. Fat is another fuel food, and part of excess protein is also available for fuel when nitrogen has been split off in the liver and converted into urea.

The value of these three foods as fuel can be estimated

by the amount of heat produced when they are burned or oxidated. This is expressed in Calories.

A large calorie is the amount of heat required to raise 1 kilogram of water 1° C.

(The small calorie used in science laboratories is the amount of heat required to raise 1 gramme of water 1° C.)

The amount of heat produced by the oxidation of the three types of food varies. Fat produces most heat, because it contains more carbon, but it needs to be burned with sugar, otherwise ketones are produced. The calorie values are:

1 ounce of protein produces 116 calories.
1 ounce of carbohydrate produces 116 calories.
1 ounce of fat produces 263 calories.

In the metric system:

1 gramme of protein produces 4·1 calories.
1 gramme of carbohydrate produces 4·1 calories.
1 gramme of fat produces 9·3 calories.

Metabolic Rate (M.R.) is the term used to express the rate at which the cells of the body work and burn sugar and oxygen. It varies in different people, depending on their activity (which is controlled largely by the thyroid gland) and their occupation.

Metabolic rate is at its lowest when all cells are at rest except those that must work to keep the body alive —the heart, blood vessels and respiratory organs. This is known as the **Basal Metabolic Rate (B.M.R.).** The B.M.R. of an individual is measured by calculation of the amount of oxygen he uses and of carbon dioxide he produces in a given time, when in bed, at rest, and fasting.

If the result is normal, it is estimated that for tissue life alone a person weighing 10 stones (63 kilograms) would require about 1,500 to 2,000 calories in twenty-four hours.

All food taken beyond this supplies the energy needed for work; and muscle activity needs a large supply of calories. The following figures are approximate only, since investigators differ in their opinions, and factors such as age, climate and the needs of the individual cause wide variations.

OCCUPATION		CALORIES REQUIRED
Active man or woman {	Heavy work ..	4,000 or more daily
	Moderate work ..	3,000 ,, ,, ,,
	Light work ..	2,500 ,, ,, ,,
	In bed	1,800 ,, ,, ,,
Growing child (12 years or over)		3,000 ,, ,, ,,

Balanced Diet. The proportion of the types of food needed varies with age and circumstances.

Protein. A large proportion should be in the form of animal protein. For adults doing light or moderate work it is considered that rather more than one-tenth of the necessary calories should be provided by protein. Growing children, expectant and nursing mothers need a much higher proportion of the total calories in the form of protein.

Fat is a valuable energy food and should provide about a quarter of the calories (including fat used in cooked foods). Since the calorie value of fat is high the actual weight and bulk needed is not great.

Carbohydrate makes up the rest of the energy food needed and the requirement varies with age, weight, work and general metabolism.

Protective foods. Foods containing all the vitamins must be included daily in the diet.

If the foods are well chosen they will contain all

necessary *mineral salts*—sodium chloride, salts of lime, phosphorus, sulphur, iron, etc.

There must also be sufficient *roughage* and plenty of *water*.

MILK

The study of the subject of milk may be made under the following headings:

A. Composition of Milk.

B. Clean Milk.

C. Safe Milk.

D. Attested Herds.

E. Tuberculin Tested Milk.

F. Heat Treated Milk:
   (*a*) Pasteurized.
   (*b*) Sterilized.

The quality of the milk produced in any country is a matter of great concern. In countries that specialise in dairy produce, such as Denmark and New Zealand, the fat content is of primary importance. In Britain most of the milk produced is sold as liquid, the remainder being used for the manufacture of National Dried Milk, and a small proportion for making cheese.

The primary concern is for the needs of infants, children and expectant and nursing mothers.

Much work is done by various bodies, including research institutes, milk marketing boards and the larger dairy companies in advising producers how to improve the quality of their milk.

It is found that in winter, and until the herds go out to pasture, there is a decline in the composition of milk, particularly in the percentage of solids-not-fat. This may be due in part to poor winter feeding, the herds needing more protein and carbohydrate in proportion to roughage.

A. Composition of Milk

The composition of milks as estimated by the Milk Marketing Board, is as follows:

Per cent.

Fat	3·56
Protein (caseinogen and lactalbumin)	3·5
Sugar	4·5
Salts (calcium, phosphorus, etc.)	0·7

Total Solids-not-fat 8·7

Vitamins

Fat-soluble A and D.

Water-soluble B_1, B_2 and C.

The remaining 87 per cent. is water.

The specific gravity is 1,030.

The reaction is faintly alkaline on milking, but soon becomes faintly acid.

The calorie value is 20 Calories for each ounce.

The Solids.

Proteins. Caseinogen is acted on in the stomach by rennin and, combining with calcium, forms a firm clot (calcium caseinate).

From three-quarters to four-fifths of milk protein is caseinogen.

The other protein, lactalbumin, does not form curds and is therefore more easily digested. It has a higher nutritive value.

Sugar. The sugar is lactose.

Salts. These, especially compounds of calcium and phosphorus for building body tissues, are present in sufficient quantities.

$Total$
$solids$ $\left\{\begin{array}{l}\text{Protein}\\\text{Sugar}\\\text{Calcium and phos-}\\\text{phorus}\\\text{Vitamin A and the B}\\\text{group}\end{array}\right\}$ The minimum standard is considered to be 8·5 per cent.

The present average is 8·7 per cent., which is satisfactory, but there are herds which produce milk that fails to reach this standard. Where this is so efforts are made to improve the winter feeding of the herds.

Fat.

The fine fat droplets are suspended in milk and, on standing, they rise to the top in the form of cream. The average fat content in England is 3·56 per cent., but in milk from Channel Island herds fat is between 4 and 5 per cent. or more.

A comparison of human milk with cows' milk shows certain differences, due largely to the different rates of growth of a baby and a calf. The following points are important:

Protein. Cows' milk contains double the total amount. The proportion of caseinogen to the more digestible lactalbumin is about 4 to 1 in cows' milk, and 2 to 1 or less in human.

The curds that form in the stomach are much tougher from cows' milk than the fine curds of human milk.

Fat. The amounts are about equal.

Sugar. Human milk contains more.

Mineral Salts are adequate in both milks. Human milk contains rather less calcium and phosphorus, and rather more iron.

Vitamins. The addition of vitamin C is considered advisable with both milks, and vitamin D in winter with cows' milk.

B. Clean Milk

Milk, *as drawn* from a healthy cow, contains comparatively few bacteria, and if hygienic methods are followed in the cowshed the milk produced will have a low bacterial count and be of a good keeping quality. Dirty milk, produced in unhygienic premises, will contain millions of bacteria, including many coliform bacilli from manure on the flanks of ungroomed cows, and will be contaminated with dust and dirt.

The "Milk and Dairies Regulations" issued by the Ministry of Agriculture gives details of the essentials for the production of clean milk. The chief requirements are summarized below.

The Cowshed or Milking House.

Site and Access. The cowshed should not be near any privy, cesspit, pig-sties or manure heap. Outside the shed there should be a concrete yard sloping to a drain inlet for easy cleaning.

Floor. This is of concrete with standings for the cows (one or both sides), with dung channels and a wide gangway. The standings are of a suitable length so that the dung will fall into the dung channels which slope slightly towards the gangway and lengthwise towards the drain outside the shed so that fluid may drain away.

Walls. These are cemented and have a smooth, washable finish up to 5 feet and above that point they are lime-washed or treated with a washable cement-paint.

Roof. The undersides of the roof should be kept free from dust by spray-washing.

Stall Divisions. These are made of smooth-faced concrete, or tubular iron, for easy cleaning and disinfection.

Lighting. Plenty of window space is necessary and the hopper type of window is the best. Good artificial light is important for milking, either a large number of 150-watt lamps, or fluorescent strip lighting.

Ventilation. The air must be kept fresh, and good ventilation is essential. Outlets should be high. Hopper windows are useful.

Feeding Troughs. These are separate for each cow and are often of glazed earthenware. Hay-racks cause contamination of the air by dust.

Water Supply. This must be plentiful. It is laid on inside the cowshed and is needed for drinking (each cow has a separate drinking bowl), for hosing the floor and dung channels, for grooming the cows and for the milkers' hand-washing. It must be kept free from contamination. There is a washbasin with soap, nailbrush and towel for the milkers.

Drainage. Liquid and dung fall into the dung channel which leads through the end wall of the cowshed. Outside the liquid flows through a grid in a trapped gully and into a drain which carries it into a concrete manure tank as far distant as possible. The tank has a cover and a pump for periodic emptying on to the land.

The dung is removed from the cowshed twice daily (but not just before milking), and carted away to the manure heap or "dungstead" which should be as far away as possible, and suitably near the tank into which the liquid can drain. A roof should protect it from rain.

Cleaning. This is most important. After removal of the dung the floor of the cowshed is cleaned, swept, and hosed down. In order to avoid contamination of the milk with dust no hay or bedding may be moved within half an hour of milking.

Milking.

The Cows. These must be thoroughly healthy. They must also be clean. Long hairs on flanks and udders are clipped and the flanks are well groomed using stiff brushes, cloths and plenty of hot water. The udders are washed carefully before each milking.

The Milkers. All milking staff must wear clean overalls and milking caps and must wash and dry their hands before milking each cow. If any milker has been in contact with a notifiable disease the dairy farmer must notify the Medical Officer of Health.

Milking. *Hand Milking.* The stools used must be scrubbed daily. The pail has a small opening placed obliquely to lessen the risk of contamination by dust. The milker's hands must be dry.

Machine Milking. This has advantages. Neither dirt from the cow nor contamination from the milker's hands can enter the milk. The clusters of teat cups, which are made of aluminium, are attached to the lid of the bucket by a short length of rubber or plastic tubing and there is a minimum of rubber piping to the pump which is worked by an electric motor in such a way that the milk is withdrawn by pressure and suction resembling the action of a calf's mouth. The milk is carried to the dairy in covered pails.

The Dairy.

In the dairy the milk is strained and cooled, and equipment is washed and sterilized.

Straining. This is done in order to remove visible dirt (not bacteria). The milk is strained through a sterile cotton wool pad resting on a perforated plate. If production has been clean there should be no dirt left on the pads.

Cooling. This is done without delay in order to check the growth of bacteria, so preventing souring and prolonging the keeping quality. Milk must be cooled to below 50° F., and preferably to 40° F. There are many types of coolers. A simple model consists of continuous tubes arranged horizontally in which cold water or brine circulates. Over this the milk flows from the top to the bottom and into the churn below. There are other more complicated refrigeration plants using other refrigerants.

Cleaning and Sterilization of Equipment. This is a most important part of clean milk production. Every vessel and appliance used must go through three stages:

(1) thorough rinsing in cold water;
(2) washing (with or without detergents);
(3) sterilizing, usually by means of steam, although boiling water or a solution of hypochlorite may be used.

Steam sterilization is carried out in a sterilizing chest for at least ten minutes.

Storage must then be in a clean place safe from contamination.

Milking machines are dismantled after milking and washed and sterilized in the same way.

Transport.

Milk is conveyed from the farms to depôts or dairies in bottles (if bottled on the farm) or in churns. Further transport may be in tanks.

Churns. These must have well fitting lids and be sealed and dated at the farm. They are collected from the farmer, often from roadside stands, where they should be sheltered from the sun, and taken to the depôts or dairies. Here the milk is cooled again and either filled into tanks for further transport, or pasteurized, or bottled. Churns should have a cold rinse and then be sterilized by steam.

Tanks. These may travel by road or be attached to trains. They are cylindrical in shape and made of either stainless steel, aluminium or glass-enamelled steel. They are insulated with cork reinforced with cement or other insulating substance. There should be no delay in transit.

Distribution.

Milk is distributed either in churns with well fitting lids, labelled and dated as described above, or in bottles which are capped and labelled either at the farm or dairy.

Milk in the Home.

In the home care should still be taken to keep the milk cool and clean either in a refrigerator or ventilated dairy. It should remain in the bottle until it is needed and after the cap is removed the top of the bottle should be wiped. The bottle should be kept covered and, in hot weather, may be stood in cold water covered with wet muslin if there is no refrigerator.

Bottles and jugs, after being emptied, should be rinsed in cold water and then washed in hot water.

C. Safe Milk

(Safe Milk implies Freedom from Pathogenic Bacteria)

Bacteria in Milk.

Non-pathogenic Bacteria. These are always present in large numbers in milk. Of these, the lactic acid bacillus is useful since it produces an acid reaction (sours the milk) so preventing the growth of putrefying bacteria which would develop in an alkaline medium, producing toxins and dangerously contaminating the milk.

This can happen to pasteurized milk, since heat treatment kills the souring bacillus but not the putrefying organisms which are sporing types.

Pathogenic bacteria may be present in milk, and can, unless the milk is heat-treated, spread the following diseases:

(*a*) From the cow:

   Tuberculosis.

   Streptococcal infections (causing sore throat or in babies, enteritis).

   Abortus fever (causing undulant fever in humans).

(*b*) From the milker:

   Diphtheria.

   Typhoid fever.

   Streptococcal infections.

   The milker may be a carrier, and he must have been careless about the rules for hygienic milking with regard to gowns, masks, hands, etc.

(*c*) From utensils such as pails, filters, bottles, etc., washed with polluted water or otherwise contaminated during or after milking, and imperfectly sterilized:

   Typhoid fever.

   Streptococcal infections.

Bacterium coli. A certain number of these bacteria in the milk is to be expected, but a heavy increase is a danger signal. Either the cows are not kept clean, or there is contamination of the water used for washing pails, etc., with sewage. Wells and drains should be investigated.

Surgical Tuberculosis. This may affect glands, bones and joints, and is caused by the bovine type of the tubercle bacillus which is present in the milk of cows with tuberculous infection. Among children the incidence, which was formerly very high, has been reduced by four-fifths since tuberculin-tested and heat-treated milks have been available.

7

Provision of a Safe Milk Supply.

In order to ensure a safe milk supply (1) dairy farmers are encouraged to own **attested herds** (see below), and (2) raw milk from all herds (except grades (*c*) and (*f*) below) undergoes heat treatment in the form of *pasteurization*.

Grading of milk is made under the following designations, and these grades cover all the milk sold in this country:

(*a*) Ordinary (pasteurized)
(*b*) Tuberculin tested (pasteurized)
(*c*) Tuberculin tested
(*d*) Channel Islands (pasteurized)
(*e*) Tuberculin tested Channel Islands (pasteurized)
(*f*) Tuberculin tested Channel Islands (farm bottled)

Licences are granted for the various grades provided that the necessary conditions are observed.

Channel Island milk contains a high percentage of fat, an average of not less than 4 per cent., and generally much higher. The producer receives a premium, and the price to the consumer is increased.

D. Attested Herds

Every encouragement is given to dairy farmers to own Attested Herds; moreover a herd must be attested before it can qualify to be a Tuberculin-Tested Herd.

If a dairy farmer wishes his herd to be attested the procedure must be as follows:

(*a*) He must produce a veterinary surgeon's certificate that no reactors to the tuberculin test were found in the herd on the last two tests made at intervals of not less than 60 days and not more than 12 months (the last test having been made within 12 months).

(*b*) The Ministry's official test will then be made on all animals in the herd.

(*c*) If no reactors are found at this test *the herd is registered* as an "Attested Herd".

Should reactors be found they must be isolated from the herd and all premises and utensils must be thoroughly disinfected. Meanwhile the herd is declared a *Supervised Herd,* and the non-reactors undergo further official tests at intervals of 60 days until no reactors are disclosed. The herd may then be registered as Attested.

Rules to be observed by the owner of an Attested Herd include the following:

(1) The Minister must be satisfied that the management of the herd and the conditions under which it is kept are suitable.

(2) A register and a record of every animal in the herd must be kept, giving descriptions, numbers and identification marks.

(3) No other cattle may enter attested premises.

(4) Fences must be kept in good repair. Usually double fencing is required.

(5) The animals may not be moved without a permit.

(6) No B.C.G. vaccination of the herd is allowed.

(7) No animal may be submitted to a tuberculin test without the consent of the Minister.

(8) An inspector from the Ministry may at any time examine the animals in the herd, the premises and the records.

The producer receives a bonus of 2*d.* a gallon for milk sold from the herd.

E. Tuberculin Tested Milk

A dairy farmer who wishes to supply milk of this special designation must obtain a T.T. licence for his herd. These licences are granted subject to special conditions and are valid for five years, after which they must be renowed.

The following are important special conditions to be observed:

(1) *The herd must be an Attested Herd.* (This became compulsory on October 1st 1954.)

This implies the observance of all rules required for attestation.

(2) Every animal in the herd must be submitted to an examination by a veterinary inspector at such times as may be required by the Minister of Agriculture.

(3) Any animal showing evidence of disease must be removed from the herd.

(4) The herd must be completely isolated from all other cattle.

(5) The producer must give to the veterinary inspector any assistance required for the purpose of a tuberculin test or examination of the animals.

(6) Methods of production, handling, storage treatment and distribution must be so operated as to comply with the provisions contained in the Milk and Dairies Regulations. (See p. 188.)

(7) *The milk*, immediately after production, must be *cooled* to a temperature not exceeding 50° F. It is then either:

(*a*) placed in *bottles* (previously steam sterilized) by the producer. Each bottle must be tightly closed with an overlapping cap which bears the address of the farm and the words "*Tuberculin Tested Milk*". There may also be added: The name of the producer; the date; the words "morning" or "evening" and the words "Farm Bottled"; or

(*b*) placed in unventilated sealed *bulk containers* labelled with the address of the farm, the date, "morning" or "evening" or "mixed milk" and the words "Tuberculin Tested Milk".

(8) Samples of the milk may be taken at any time and tested in the milk-testing laboratory. They must satisfy the prescribed test.

Tuberculin Tested milk is tubercle-free, but it is not necessarily free from other pathogenic bacteria. For that reason, when used for infants, it is usually either pasteurized, when it is labelled "*Tuberculin Tested Milk (Pasteurized)*", or sterilized when it is labelled "*Tuberculin Tested Milk (Sterilized)*".

Producers of Tuberculin Tested milk receive a premium of 4*d*. per gallon.

F. Heat Treatment

This may be either Pasteurization or Sterilization.

PASTEURIZATION

The High Temperature Short Time (H.T.S.T.) "Paraflow" System.

The milk arrives at the dairy in milk cans and is tipped into—

1. **Tipping Tanks** and is then pumped to a—

2. **Balance Tank,** which is float-controlled (in large dairies there are insulated stainless steel storage tanks). The milk then passes through a flow controller to the—

3. **Heat Exchanger.** Here the milk is **pre-heated** as it flows through tubes (or grooved plates) adjacent to other tubes containing the *hot* milk returning from the holder (see No. 6). Thus the raw milk is pre-heated and the returning milk is cooled ("heat-exchange"). It then passes through—

4. **A Filter** and back to—

5. **The Heater** where the temperature is raised to 161° F. The milk then enters—

6. **The Holding Section.** This is contained in the lower part of the control panel. The milk passes through in **15 seconds, held at a temperature of 161° F.** The illustration at the end of the book is of a tubular type. The tube is made of stainless steel and is air-insulated. At the inlet is the bulb of a thermometer to record the tempera-

ture, combined with a "flow-diversion" valve to divert any milk that is not entering at the correct temperature. The milk, *now pasteurized*, passes out of the holding tube and back through—

7. The Water-and-Brine Cooling Section (in the heat-exchanger) where the temperature is reduced to 40° F. The milk passes on to—

8. Bottling and Capping machines, each of which can fill and cap over 100 bottles a minute. The caps are marked "*Pasteurized Milk*" or if T.T. "*Tuberculin Tested Milk (Pasteurized)*". The bottles are then taken to—

9. The Cold Store where the temperature is kept at 38°–40° F.

All tubes in the equipment are of stainless steel, and the plant takes up little room, one "Paraflow" dealing with 2000–3000 gallons an hour.

An Older Method of Pasteurization.

This method is in use in some dairies. The filtered, pre-heated milk is filled into a *Holder* which is a large revolving container divided into compartments that are insulated from the outer jacket. The milk enters at *a temperature* of 145°–150° F. and is held at that temperature *for 30 minutes*, after which it is discharged and immediately *cooled to 50° F.*

In large dairies there are usually two laboratories. In one incoming milk is tested for (*a*) keeping quality, (*b*) fat content, and (*c*) solids-not-fat content. In the other, frequent samples of the pasteurized milk are tested, with the object of discovering whether pasteurization has been efficient.

The Methylene Blue Test indicates the purity of the milk. If the samples decolorize quickly there is an excessive number of bacteria present.

The Phosphatase Test. There is an enzyme in milk, phosphatase, which should be destroyed by heat treatment. If it is present in samples, pasteurization is not complete.

Other Methods of Pasteurization.

In Children's Hospitals. The milk for baby feeds for twenty-four hours is in measure bottles in a cruet stand. These are kept at the correct temperature for the required time in steam sterilizers, the same bottles being used for feeding.

For household use a double saucepan may be used. The water in the outer pan should boil for two minutes. This is not an accurate method.

Results of Pasteurization.

Milk is made safe since all pathogenic organisms are destroyed. Many non-pathogenes are also destroyed, including the souring bacilli. There is very slight precipitation of lactalbumin, calcium and phosphates (not more than 5 per cent.).

Vitamins A, B_2 and D are not affected.

Vitamin B_1 is slightly reduced.

Vitamin C is reduced by rather less than one-third in the H.T.S.T. method.

STERILIZATION

The milk is filtered, homogenized (*i.e.* the fat globules are emulsified so that fat is uniformly distributed) and it is then subjected to heat treatment at a **temperature of 212° F.** Bottling is done after boiling, and on completion the bottles are sealed with an airtight seal.

The labels are marked "*Sterilized Milk*" or "*Tuberculin Tested Milk (Sterilized)*" as the case may be.

Samples are tested in the laboratory for turbidity. If the test is satisfactory the milk will show no turbidity.

This milk is absolutely *safe* for infants. There is some precipitation of the protein lactalbumin but it does not, as when milk is boiled, coagulate and form a "skin" which has to be removed.

Vitamin C is reduced, but fruit juice will compensate for this.

Milk *in the home* may be boiled and is then quite safe for infants. The coagulated lactalbumin ("skin") should be given separately (flavoured) as it is a valuable protein.

Dried Milk

All water is evaporated and bacteria are destroyed. Vitamin C may sometimes be reduced; but it is claimed that the roller process does not destroy it. In any case it is never very plentiful in milk, and every baby should be given orange juice or other fruit juice.

Methods. (1) *Roller Process.* A thin film of milk is fed on to revolving heated rollers at a temperature just under boiling-point. In three seconds the water is evaporated, and the milk falls in fine flakes into containers.

(2) *Spray Process.* Milk is sprayed into a hot-air chamber and falls on the floor as a fine powder, the water being immediately evaporated.

National Full Cream Dried Milk. This is prepared by the roller process. It has a high fat content.

National Half Cream Dried Milk. This has had some of the fat removed. Both these milks are reconstituted by adding one drachm of powder to one ounce of water.

Proprietary Dried Milks have been modified in various ways to make them more digestible or more like human milk. Dried milks are sterile and keep well, but are deficient in vitamin C.

Evaporated Milk. This has had water evaporated from it till it is one-third of its former bulk. It is sterile when the tin is opened, but is easily infected by flies, spoons, etc., and it will not keep.

("Food-borne diseases" and "Keeping of food", see Chapter XII.)

CHAPTER XII

FOOD CONTAMINATION AND PRESERVATION

CARE OF FOOD IN THE HOME

Contamination.

DANGEROUS contamination of food is due to **bacteria.**
Food is organic substance, and is therefore an excellent
medium for the growth of bacteria, provided there is
moisture, a suitable temperature and, usually, air.

Some organisms are already present in food, and
these types will cause decomposition unless the food
has been subjected to proper treatment followed by
suitable methods of storage. Other types are introduced
into the food during preparation or serving. Infection
of food is the cause of either (*a*) food-borne diseases or
(*b*) food poisoning.

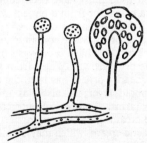

FIG. 66.—THE PIN-MOULD (MUCOR).

Moulds.

These are fungi, and many types attack food, growing
on jam, fruit, bread, etc. They spread by spores, which

7*

fall on food from the air or are carried by flies, and the growth, once started, spreads rapidly, the spores being scattered around. They spoil food, making it unfit for eating, though the substances they produce are not actually toxic.

Yeasts.

These cause fermentation, converting starch to glucose and glucose to alcohol, carbon dioxide and water. Yeast cells are present in the air and are obtained by culture.

Food-borne Diseases.

The bacteria of **typhoid** and **paratyphoid fever** (belonging to the Salmonella group) and the bacilli of **dysentery** when taken in through the mouth in infected food, set up inflammation in the intestines, and are passed out in the stools. After recovery the patient may still harbour the organisms for years, continuing to pass them in his stools. He has thus become a **carrier** and may be the cause of a succession of cases of the disease until he is discovered by laboratory tests on the stools.

The infected food must have been contaminated by excreta from a carrier or from a patient with the active disease. The infection may be conveyed to the food by unwashed hands, or by water contaminated by sewage effluent in which salads have been washed, or in which watercress has been grown. Water from shallow wells infected from nearby privies has been the cause of outbreaks of typhoid fever; so also has milk from unhygienic dairy farms. Numbers of outbreaks have been traced to ice-cream handled by carriers, and many again to synthetic cream, which may be infected during the process of filling cakes, or selling them in the retail shop.

Milk-borne Diseases.

These have been discussed in Chapter XI.

Food Poisoning.

Numbers of outbreaks of food poisoning occur every year, sometimes affecting groups of people as in families, schools, canteens, etc. and, at other times, involving widespread areas where the infected food has been distributed from factories. Patients are usually taken suddenly, and often violently ill.

The types of organisms that cause food poisoning are four in number, of which three are intestinal bacteria.

Salmonella. This is a big group of intestinal bacteria, some varieties of which are the commonest cause of food poisoning. They infect animals, and the contaminated carcases may further infect other meat in slaughter-house or shop. Outbreaks are usually due to meat that has been partly cooked and then re-cooked, the bacilli having multiplied in the interval. Rats and mice are very susceptible to Salmonella infection and are a source of danger in food premises. Ducks may also be infected, in which case their eggs would contain the bacteria.

Within 24 hours of eating the infected food, the patient is taken ill with vomiting, diarrhoea and colic.

Clostridium welchii—Clostridium botulinum. These are also intestinal organisms. They are sporebearers and anærobes but, fortunately, they are both rare. If they are present in meat or vegetables any food left over and eaten later would be dangerous as the spores are not killed by cooking and the organisms would have developed and multiplied in the interval.

Clostridium welchii causes only mild symptoms, but **botulism** is very fatal. Symptoms appear in 24 hours or longer. The patient is giddy and collapses and in a short time paralyses develop causing double vision, inability to swallow and, when the diaphragm is affected, death often occurs.

Staphylococci. This is the fourth type of organism that causes food poisoning, but unlike the others staphylococci are not intestinal bacteria, they are pyogenic and are present in septic spots, boils, and often in the nose. They are introduced into the food by the hands of those engaged in its preparation, either directly from a septic focus, or from the nose via a handkerchief. When in the food the staphylococci produce **poisonous toxins,** and within a few hours of eating the patient collapses with vomiting, diarrhoea and abdominal pain. Recovery is rapid.

PRESERVATION OF FOOD

In order to kill bacteria food must be subjected to **heat treatment** and to preserve food indefinitely the temperature must be sufficiently high and maintained for a time sufficient to ensure that spores are destroyed. **Dehydration** is a useful method for some foods, but bacteria may become active again when the food is reconstituted.

For storage of food refrigeration is the method used.

Heat Treatment

Bacteria, except the sporing types, are killed rapidly at temperatures above 160° F. Sporing bacilli need a much higher temperature maintained for a longer time. Methods of treating food by heat are based on intensive research in order to find the best means of ensuring its safety and preserving its flavour.

Methods in Use:

1. **Pasteurization of Milk.** See p. 197.
2. **Boiling.** This method is used for preserving fruit, with the addition of sugar.
3. **Canning.** This is suitable for meat, fish, vegetables and fruit. Tins are filled with the food partly cooked,

and fitted with lids in which a hole is left. All the air is then sucked out through this hole and the tins are sealed. They are then heated in an autoclave to a temperature, which varies and may be up to 250° F. in order to destroy bacteria and their spores. After this they are cooled rapidly. Any bacteria not killed would, by decomposing the food, produce gas which would bulge the ends of the tin, and liquid which would be heard on shaking the tin. Such tins are called "blown tins" and should not be used.

Dehydration

Meat, fish, eggs, milk, vegetables and fruit may be dehydrated. Water is removed from the food, usually by some process of heating, and this renders it unsuitable for growth of bacteria, since they need moisture. If the drying process is complete, as in dried eggs and milk, etc., no further treatment is necessary, but meat and fish often need salting or smoking in addition.

Dried fruits are also preserved by the sugar they contain.

Preservative Substances

(a) **Smoking and Salting.** These processes are used for fish and meat. Either process may be used, or they may be combined, in which case the food is soaked in brine first and then hung for a few days in the smoke of smouldering oak, the fumes of which contain creosote.

(b) **Other Chemical Substances.** Certain other substances are allowed to be used for preserving in specified quantities.

Cold Storage

The transport of food from one country to another, even through the tropics, is made possible by cold storage. Meat, fish, butter, fruit, etc., are carried in this way, and after landing are kept in large cold stores until needed.

Cold such as is used for preserving meat is not sufficiently intense to kill all bacteria, but their growth and activity are inhibited. When the meat is taken out of the store and brought up to normal temperature, the bacteria and other organisms regain their activity and act on the meat.

(NOTE. Certain fungi are capable of remaining active even in these cold rooms, and may give rise to the condition of "black spot" and "whiskers" on meat.)

Cold storage is made possible by the fact that rapid evaporation of a liquid requires heat to be taken from the surroundings, that is, it has a cooling effect.

Household Refrigerators.

These are of different patterns but all work on the same principle—that a liquid evaporating into a gas takes heat from the surroundings in the cabinet so reducing the temperature.

Outside the cabinet (at the back or underneath, and enclosed) is an electric motor working a compressor pump attached to a compressor coil. In this coil the refrigerant gas is compressed into liquid which passes up a pipe and through a valve into the cooling coil inside the cabinet. Here the liquid evaporates into a gas, taking the heat needed for the process from the air and food and from the water in the ice-box which freezes into cubes of ice. The gas passes back by another pipe to the compressor coil, again to be compressed into a liquid, repeating the circuit continuously. A refrigerant in general use is a chemical that goes under various trade names ("Freon", etc.) while some make use of ammonia and hydrogen.

In some cases the motor is run by gas.

Insulation. It is necessary to insulate all cold chambers from the surrounding air. The hollow jacket which surrounds the inner chamber is filled with pressed granulated cork or glass wool.

Large Cold Storage Rooms.

The refrigerant used is liquid ammonia with the addition of hydrogen to increase the cooling effect. The evaporation into ammonia gas takes place in a cooling coil in a tank of brine, the gas being condensed into liquid again in another coil. The cold brine from the tank circulates in pipes round the storeroom, returning to the tank for re-cooling. The temperatures required in the storerooms are:

For "frozen" meat 10°–15° F.
For "chilled" meat 28°–30° F.
For fruit a variable temperature above freezing point depending on the type of fruit.

Ice is not of much practical value for preserving food. Ice boxes were used before other means of refrigeration were available.

Solid Carbon Dioxide. This is a very useful refrigerant for some purposes. It is employed in ice cream containers, and also to preserve fruit during long transport. In addition to its intense cooling power, it slowly evaporates, becoming carbon dioxide gas which, in suitable quantities, acts as a further preservative.

Quick- or Deep-Freezing. This is the latest method of preserving food by cold. The foods are first treated to destroy enzyme action, and then sealed in cellophane-lined packets which go into the quick-freezing tunnel at a temperature sometimes as low as −5° F. With this rapid penetration of cold the food retains its original freshness. These "frosted foods" have to be used quickly, even if they are kept in a refrigerator.

Keeping Food in the Home.

A *refrigerator*, as described above, is the only really satisfactory means. If this is not possible there are various devices which serve to keep food cool, depending on the fact that water will soak up through a porous substance which must be so placed as to surround the food.

Butter coolers, milk coolers, and even a small type of "cooling cabinet" work on this principle.

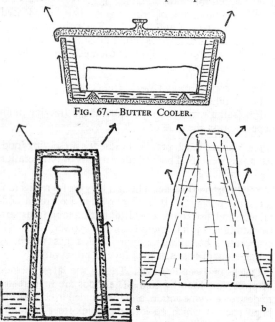

FIG. 67.—BUTTER COOLER.

FIG. 68.—TWO MILK COOLERS.

Figs. 67 and 68 illustrate some of these. In Fig. 68B wet muslin takes the place of the wet porous pot.

CONTAMINATION OF FOOD

Intensive investigations are carried out every time an outbreak of **food poisoning** or **food-borne disease** occurs. The case is notified to the Medical Officer of Health and every effort is made to trace the source.

Any remains of the suspected food are examined in the laboratory to discover the organism.

Samples of vomit and stools are collected from all who have been taken ill, and swabs from the nose and hands of all who have handled the food, as well as stool samples if the organism is an intestinal type. Food factories and kitchens are visited and swabs are taken from tables, implements and utensils. Sanitary Inspectors leave no stone unturned in their efforts to discover the cause.

Any health visitor or nurse who happens to be present where there is suspected food poisoning before the doctor arrives, should see that all food left over is kept and that all vomit and stools from the patients are saved.

Food that May be the Cause of Outbreaks.

The most frequent cause is contamination of some form of meat food. Infection of carcases with Salmonella is not obvious on inspection. One infected animal, through handling in slaughter-house or shop, may be responsible for infection of other meat.

Reheated Meat Dishes. These are a source of danger on account of spore forming organisms. Should these be present the spores would not be killed by the first cooking, and would develop and multiply in the interval, unless the food was kept in a refrigerator.

Meat Pies and Sausages. Both these have been the cause of outbreaks due to undercooking. The centre needs to reach a high temperature as well as the outside.

Meat Rolls and other types of *Processed Meat*. These may be infected by handling during preparation. A worker with a septic abrasion on his hand has been known to infect the food with staphylococci which, in a medium so favourable, produced dangerous toxins, causing outbreaks of food poisoning wherever the meat was sold.

Ducks' Eggs. These are very occasionally found to contain Salmonella. Although duck may be infected with the organism, hens' eggs are exempt. Ducks' eggs should be used only in dishes cooked at a high temperature.

Ice Cream. Outbreaks of typhoid and paratyphoid fever have recurred at intervals due usually to carriers and unhygienic methods of food preparation and storage. In 1947 legislation was introduced by which the mixture, after the heating process, must be frozen immediately and kept frozen until it is sold. In this way organisms, if present, would not develop. Sanitary Inspectors visit premises to see that these regulations are carried out.

Synthetic Cream. Cakes, buns, meringues, etc. filled with synthetic cream have accounted for a large number of outbreaks of typhoid and paratyphoid fever. The cream is liable to be handled, either in the bakery or in the shop, and the infection may be conveyed by a carrier. All utensils used for filling should be sterilized, and cakes should be handled with tongs—not hands.

Fish. Fresh or frozen are safe unless processed and subjected to handling. Oysters may be infected with typhoid and paratyphoid bacteria due to sewage contamination of the shallow sea bed where they are grown.

Cured Meat and Cured Fish. These, if kept dry, are safe for a considerable time.

The Food and Drugs Act, 1938

This Act lays down laws concerning premises where food is prepared or sold. By it also food poisoning is made notifiable. In 1949 further regulations by means of Bye-laws dealt in detail with the handling and wrapping of food, protection from dust, animals, etc., disposal of refuse and other matters concerning food hygiene.

More recently the Ministry of Food has published the findings resulting from investigation into the conduct of catering establishments and food hygiene in general, and further legislation is now before Parliament.

Premises Used for Handling Food

Slaughter-houses. These are licensed and inspected, and humane killing is enforced.

All carcases are inspected, and many hundreds of tons of meat are condemned every year as being unfit for food, due to obvious diseases such as tuberculosis, "measly" condition, etc. Occasionally it may happen that meat may be infected with Salmonella organisms from the intestine of an animal that is a healthy carrier.

Transport of meat is not at present always up to the desired standard.

Factories. In premises where food is prepared and processed a high level of hygiene should be maintained. Pressed meat, pies, brawns and sausage may easily be infected at some stage in their manufacture due to handling, contaminated utensils, etc.

Gelatin is a specially good medium for the growth of bacteria if after being infected it remains at a warm temperature.

Retail Shops. Food should not be exposed where customers can handle it and cough over it. In butchers' and fishmongers' refrigerated show-cases should be installed and, in pastry cooks', glass screens should be fitted where food is displayed. Cakes and pastries should not be handled at all. The tongs that are provided for the purpose should always be **used**.

Animals should not be allowed to roam about in shops.

Kitchens and Catering Establishments. Floors and walls should be washable. Ventilation should be efficient; ducts and extraction fans being fitted over all cookers and sinks. There should be a plentiful water supply, both hot and cold, ample cloak-rooms and sanitary facilities, and good lighting.

Washing Up. In all large premises washing machines are used. There are various types and sizes. In general the washing water is about 140° F. and the rinse water 160° F. or more. Coming out of water at this temperature the articles dry quickly without the use of cloths. If washing up is done by hand the water should be equally hot, especially the rinse water which should be in a second sink or bowl. Sinks are of stainless steel and the water is heated usually by electricity and there is thermostatic control.

A good detergent should be used, and all mops and cloths should be boiled every day.

There are many good detergents on the market and most of them contain water-softening substances.

Benches, Tables and Draining Boards. These should be metal topped. Wooden benches are still in use in many premises that have not been modernized and they are most unsatisfactory since, in spite of careful cleaning, bacteria remain in cracks.

Refuse Bins. These must be kept covered and cleaned efficiently. They should be raised from the ground.

Vermin. By an Act that came into force in 1950 anyone whose premises are infested by **rats or mice** is bound to report the matter to the Local Authority and to take such steps to destroy them as shall be specified by the Authority. Not only do rats and mice devour much food every year and foul still more, but they may be infected with Salmonella, in which case their droppings are very dangerous and have been known to cause outbreaks of intestinal infection. The occupier of premises where there is vermin infestation is bound to

ensure that any possible route of entry for rodents is
blocked; that no food is left lying about; that food containers are of metal or other impervious material with
lids always kept on them. There is still the problem of
rat runs under floors from other premises, and the Local
Authority will take all necessary steps to deal with this.

Cockroaches swarm especially where there are
covered-in heating pipes. The Local Authority will use
insecticides, but may ultimately require the ducts containing hot pipes to be opened up for more efficient
treatment.

Flies. The most important measure to prevent breeding of flies is to ensure that there is no garbage or food
waste left about and also that no refuse bins are left
uncovered. To prevent contamination of food it is
essential that it should be covered. If for sale to
display, covers of glass, cellophane or perspex will
serve. For destruction of flies D.D.T. or Gammexane
sprays are good provided they are not used near food.

The Handling of Food. Those who handle food should
wear clean overalls. They should keep their nails short
and clean and wash their hands after visiting the toilet
and before starting to prepare food. They should avoid
coughing and sneezing over food and should wash their
hands after using a handkerchief. Hot air driers are
the best means of drying the hands or, failing this, the
continuous roller towel method, but on no account
should there be a communal towel. Any food handler
who has septic spots, a sore throat, or an attack of
diarrhoea and vomiting must report at once to the
manager.

It is essential to avoid touching food with the hands
whenever possible.

The Preparation of Food in the Small Home

Where food is prepared in the small home it is not
always possible to arrange a small kitchen in the ideal

way, but certain aims may be kept in mind. Food and store cupboards and food preparation benches should be on one side of the cooker, and the sink, china cupboards and service table on the other side. It is a great advantage if the tops of low cupboards, tables, cooker and sinkboards can be on the same level. The refrigerator may be the built-in type or free-standing. A low ventilated cupboard for vegetables is needed. Kitchen cabinets are useful.

The Sink Unit. This should be of stainless steel, rather than of fireclay, with hardwood drainage boards.

A small electric extraction fan in the window or outer wall will clear all smells and steam.

The hot water supply may be from a slow combustion stove (which necessitates extra cleaning) or a hot water storage tank with an immersion heater and thermostatic control.

Alternatively a small water heater can be fitted over the sink.

Preparation and service working tables should have washable surfaces.

Lighting is important. Diffused type fittings are best, and local lights may be needed over the cooker and sink.

Washing up demands a really hot water supply and a good detergent. The drying of teacloths, etc., can be made easy by fixing a rail under the draining board with a small electric tubular heater below protected with wire mesh.

CHAPTER XIII

SOCIAL SERVICES

ADMINISTRATION

THE growth and development of Public Health has advanced steadily through more than a hundred years. From about 1840 onwards there was a growing realization of the need to do something to better the appalling slum conditions in the large towns, which were the outcome of the shift of population from the country to the industrial areas. In this incredibly difficult task the early results were due to the work of individuals—men and women who in their different fields of work laboured to relieve poverty, distress and disease. The frequent epidemics of smallpox, typhoid fever, cholera and typhus fever that swept the country were responsible for a very high death rate every year, and when it was realized that the spread of these diseases was directly due to the contamination of water, and to the presence of refuse and vermin, these matters were made the subject of an Act of Parliament, and the **first Public Health Act** was passed in 1875. By this Act the country was divided up into urban and rural districts and county boroughs, each of which had a Council, which for the purposes of the Act was known as the Local Sanitary Authority. Later, the urban and rural districts were put under **County Councils** for certain health purposes, but the large towns remained complete authorities, as **County Borough Councils**. These bodies are still known as **Local Health Authorities,** and are responsible for administering the various Acts which have since been passed. These Acts were concerned with sanitary measures which would lessen the danger of outbreaks of infectious diseases and improve living conditions. They included control of sewage disposal, protection of water supplies, demolition of slum areas, prevention of nuisances, and protection of food supplies. In 1936 **the second Public Health Act** was passed. It amended and consolidated all the previous Acts, including the **Notification of Infectious Diseases Act,** and was followed later by the **Food and Drugs Act.** From 1902 onwards the social services were established and developed by a number of acts, such as the **Midwives Acts, Maternity and Child Welfare Act,** the **Children Act** and many others. During the same years **Education Acts** were passed which placed the responsibility for education in the hands of Local Authorities, and school medical services were instituted.

Gradually, in the minds of those responsible, the concept of Public Health has changed. It is not now just a question of the prevention of disease, this aspect is no less important, but is supplemented by the purpose to use every means of ensuring good health and fitness both of mind and body. This **positive aim** is the basis of all the new trends in Public Health.

It includes not only medical services, but also diet and environment, and environment covers housing, sanitation, the home, the conditions of work and education, and all that affects the standard of living.

A wide and comprehensive scheme was needed which would link up the Ministries concerned in this new concept, and in 1946 the **National Health Act** was passed. The following tables give the details of the scheme and shows where there is liaison with the **Ministries of Education** and **Housing and Local Government.**

The general structure will be seen from Tables A and B below.

TABLE A

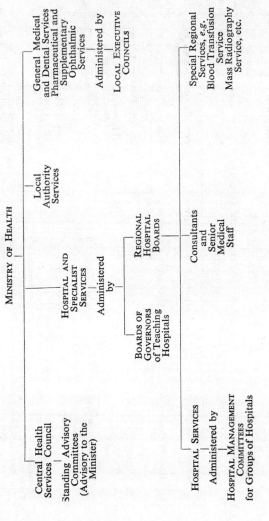

MINISTRY OF HEALTH

Central Health Services Council
Standing Advisory Committees (Advisory to the Minister)

Local Authority Services

Hospital and Specialist Services
Administered by

Boards of Governors of Teaching Hospitals

Regional Hospital Boards

Consultants and Senior Medical Staff

Special Regional Services, e.g. Blood Transfusion Service Mass Radiography Service, etc.

Hospital Services
Administered by
Hospital Management Committees for Groups of Hospitals

General Medical and Dental Services Pharmaceutical and Supplementary Ophthalmic Services
Administered by
Local Executive Councils

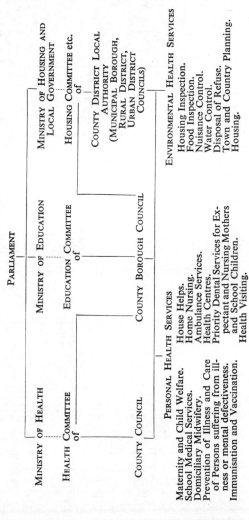

TABLE B

LOCAL AUTHORITY HEALTH SERVICES

PARLIAMENT

MINISTRY OF HEALTH	MINISTRY OF EDUCATION	MINISTRY OF HOUSING AND LOCAL GOVERNMENT
HEALTH COMMITTEE of	EDUCATION COMMITTEE of	HOUSING COMMITTEE etc. of
COUNTY COUNCIL	COUNTY BOROUGH COUNCIL	COUNTY DISTRICT LOCAL AUTHORITY (MUNICIPAL BOROUGH, RURAL DISTRICT, URBAN DISTRICT COUNCILS)

PERSONAL HEALTH SERVICES

Maternity and Child Welfare.
School Medical Services.
Domiciliary Midwifery.
Prevention of Illness and Care of Persons suffering from illness or mental defectiveness.
Immunisation and Vaccination.
House Helps.
Home Nursing.
Ambulance Services.
Health Centres.
Priority Dental Services for Expectant and Nursing Mothers and School Children.
Health Visiting.

ENVIRONMENTAL HEALTH SERVICES

Housing Inspection.
Food Inspection.
Nuisance Control.
Water Control.
Disposal of Refuse.
Town and Country Planning.
Housing.

All matters concerning the health of the people, therefore, are in the charge of a **Central Authority, the Ministry of Health.** The **Minister of Health** has as advisers a **Chief Medical Officer** and a **Chief Nursing Officer,** with assistants both professional, executive and clerical.

The Central Authority prepares and supervises the implementation of the **Acts of Parliament** which deal with all matters concerning health: these laws are then administered in all parts of the country by **Local Authorities** which are either **County Councils** or, for large towns, **County Borough Councils.** The National Health Service Act is an exception in that the hospital and general practitioner services are administered by special machinery set up for the purpose under the Act, and the public health services only are administered by the local authorities. The Health Service is financed partly from National Insurance Act Contributions, and partly from taxation.

It is intended that eventually general practitioner and local authority health services and clinics shall be grouped together in Health Centres.

The Local Health Authority has trained personnel to carry out these services.

Other central agencies concerned with health are:

1. **The Ministry of Education** concerned with the health of school children.

2. **The Ministry of National Insurance** administering the various National Insurance Acts, 1946–1952, by means of which practically everyone between school-leaving age and pensionable age pays contributions and receives various benefits, including sickness and maternity benefits, and eventually a retirement pension.

3. **The Ministry of Agriculture and Fisheries** dealing with food inspection and prevention of spread of disease in cattle.

4. **The Home Office** dealing with Industrial Hygiene and Deprived Children.

5. **The Ministry of Town and Country Planning.**

6. **The Ministry of Labour.**

7. **The Admiralty, War Office and Air Ministry** concerned with the health of the Forces.

PERSONNEL

The Medical Officer of Health is in charge of his area with one or more assistants, and a large staff of specialists which includes:

Public Health Inspectors, who are concerned with the administration of the sanitary laws;

Specialist Tuberculosis Officers
School Medical Officer
Children's Officer
Welfare Officer   } Concerned with
Health Visitors   personal services.
Midwives
Home Nurses

A large clerical staff is required in all departments.

The Medical Officer of Health

The M.O.H. is appointed by a Local Authority which may be a County Council, a County Borough Council, or an Urban or Rural District Council. He is responsible for the health service administered by the Local Authority which appoints him.

A County Medical Officer of Health is responsible for, among other things:

Maternity and Child Welfare Services.
Domiciliary Midwives' Service.
Home Nursing.
Prevention of Infection.

Vaccination and Immunization.
Ambulance Services.
Registration and Inspection of Nursing Homes.
After Care.
(Usually) School Medical Services.

The M.O.H. of a Rural or Urban District is responsible for the supervision and control of local sanitary conditions, housing conditions, nuisances, food inspection and analyses, and other duties carried out on his behalf by Sanitary Inspectors. He is responsible for the control of infectious diseases, and may have certain duties of the County Medical Officer delegated to him and be appointed and paid as a part-time member of the County Medical Officer's staff.

The County Borough Medical Officer of Health has all the duties of the County Medical Officer and the County District Medical Officer for the area of his county borough.

The Public Health Inspector

The Public Health Inspector must hold a diploma granted by certain examining and training bodies. He is required to work under the direction of the M.O.H., to inspect his district and to keep himself informed regarding the sanitary condition of the district. He is called in to investigate any complaints of insanitary conditions in houses, and to see that they are put right; he inspects verminous premises and arranges for disinfestation; he must take samples of water if there is question of pollution; he investigates dairy farms in his area, and inspects premises where food is prepared and sold, taking samples for analysis when he thinks necessary.

One or more Inspectors usually specialize in *smoke abatement*, and are made responsible for this branch of the work.

Public Health Inspectors may be men or women.

The Local Authority may approve a qualified veterinary surgeon as a Public Health Inspector for purposes connected with the inspection of meat.

Sanitary Laws.

The work of the Public Health Inspector is concerned with the practical application of the sanitary laws. These laws are incorporated in the Public Health Acts and they comprise legislation for many branches and aspects of Public Health

Their scope is very wide, and only a few main indications can be outlined here.

Dwelling Houses. The Housing Act of 1936 consolidated all previous Housing Acts. It appoints as Local Authorities responsible for administering the Act the Borough, Urban and Rural District Councils, and the London County Council. It includes laws relating to:

Repair and drainage of houses.

Demolition of unfit premises.

Clearance of large areas of unfit dwellings.

Redevelopment of these and other areas.

Prevention of overcrowding in houses.

Powers of acquiring land for new housing plans, and for provision of water and gas for the houses.

Provisions to safeguard parks, commons and open spaces.

Drainage laws relate to:

Drains and sewers, their construction, traps, ventilation, etc.

Pollution of rivers with sewage.

Construction of privies and cesspools.

Sewage disposal works.

Water-closets, their type and the number to be provided in factories.

Water. Various Acts provide that:

Every house must have a sufficient supply of pure water.

No new house may be occupied until the Sanitary Authority gives a certificate that there is a proper water supply.

If there is any complaint that a well is polluted, the water must be analysed and the well may be closed if necessary.

River water must not be polluted by sewage, factory waste, etc.

Offensive Trades. This law is designed to prevent nuisance or danger to health from odours or other effects of certain trades—*e.g.*, soap, tallow, bone, blood or tripe boilers; also chimneys emitting excessive black smoke.

Nuisances. These are any conditions injurious to health. They include badly constructed or leaking cesspools, drains and privies, rubbish dumps, excessive black smoke, etc.; such conditions must be removed by order.

Infectious Diseases. Various Acts deal with procedures such as:

Notification of certain diseases (see p. 128) to the M.O.H., who in turn notifies the County M.O.H. and the Ministry of Health.

Disinfection of premises and articles infected, including library books.

Closure of schools in some cases.

Following up of contacts.

Vaccination of children and smallpox contacts.

Clearing rats from ships (see p. 151).

Provision for treatment of venereal disease.

Cleansing of verminous persons, houses and articles.

Other Acts concerned with Food, Factories, etc., are explained later.

PERSONAL SERVICES

Welfare work is carried out in clinics, in nurseries, in various types of residential institutions, and in the homes of the people. Working in co-operation with doctors and specialists are health visitors, midwives, school and home nurses, the domestic helps and ambulance services.

Maternity Services

The Health Service provides for the expectant mother a choice of two alternatives. She may choose to have her baby at home (domiciliary service), the delivery being taken usually by a midwife or, if she prefers, by her doctor with a maternity nurse in attendance; or she may have her baby in hospital.

Under the National Health Service admission to the maternity department of a hospital is allowed for two main reasons—because there is a medical priority, or because there is a social priority, for example, a shared home or an overcrowded home. Any patient, of course, may make arrangements, at her own expense, to have her baby in a private nursing home or in the private beds of a Health Service Hospital. If there is the difficulty of leaving a young family for two weeks, this can usually be overcome with the assistance of relatives or "home helps".

In either case antenatal hygiene is of great importance. If the expectant mother decides to have her baby at home she will see her doctor at intervals, and the nurse she engages will visit and advise her. The alternative is to attend antenatal clinics.

The Antenatal Clinic.

The staff at the clinic consists of a doctor assisted by midwives. The expectant mother is seen by the doctor at her first visit and again about a month before the baby is due. She should attend also each month, when she will be seen by the midwife and, if it should be necessary, by the doctor.

At the first visit the examination will include:

> History of previous health, pregnancies, labours and puerperia.
> Pelvic measurements and abdominal examination.
> Urine testing.
> Blood pressure.

At monthly visits the midwife will take her blood pressure, test her urine, and weigh her carefully. An increase in weight above the normal is one of the first signs of toxæmia.

She will then give advice on simple points of hygiene and routine, which will help the expectant mother to meet the exigencies of pregnancy and support the strain without ill effects.

The mother has to provide both the growing fœtus and herself with the right kind and quantity of nourishment. She also has to excrete the waste products of her own metabolism and that of the fœtus, and the strain of this is thrown largely on the liver and kidneys, since these organs deal with and dispose of such products.

Diet. This is of the greatest importance. The chief points are:

Protein is needed for cell building, and should be taken two or three times a week in normal amounts, especially animal protein in meat, fish, eggs, cheese and milk.

Fruit and vegetables should be eaten as much as possible and especially raw, as in salads. This will provide the salts needed by the growing fœtus, and roughage to prevent constipation.

Bread should be wholemeal, and porridge is good.

Milk. If possible two pints a day should be drunk. One pint is allowed at a reduced price. Butter also should be included in the diet.

8

Fluids should be taken freely to assist the kidneys to excrete waste products. Milk drinks, fruit drinks and water are all valuable.

Vitamins. Protective foods are most important, and although the diet outlined contains them all, the expectant mother needs cod-liver oil, orange juice and Marmite or alternatively vitamin capsules, to supplement the diet.

At the clinic she will be given free cod-liver oil or Multivite tablets and concentrated orange juice at a low price.

The daily meals should include meat or fish or cheese, milk, butter, eggs, plenty of vegetables, fruit and salad, brown bread or porridge, and several pints of fluid. No food likely to upset the digestion should be taken.

Clothing. The problem of abdominal support is of first importance. This should be support without compression, and for some months can be provided by corsets which should be sufficiently elastic and should give support from below. Later an abdominal belt or binder may be worn instead. A breast support (not brassière) may also be needed. There must be no constriction to the circulation, such as garters, and nothing should interfere with breathing.

High heels should not be worn, because they throw out the normal balance of the body and hinder free walking. Excess clothes should be avoided.

The Bowels. A regular daily action is necessary, since constipation causes toxæmia which may have serious results. Plenty of fruit, vegetables, brown bread or porridge, and water to drink, may keep the bowels acting so long as daily exercise is possible. Otherwise mild aperients such as cascara or infusion of senna pods should be taken.

Teeth. Carious teeth are a real danger. They may provide a focus from which toxins are continuously poured into the circulation, causing various toxic conditions. The mother will be advised to have such teeth extracted, and to pay great attention to daily cleaning of the mouth and teeth.

Baths. Daily warm baths should be taken all through pregnancy, and if that is not possible, a sponge all over should take its place, since, by this means, the skin is kept functioning well.

The Breasts. These should be washed daily with soap and water and dried, but massage and other treatment is not advisable. Supports may be worn if necessary. Special care should be taken of the nipples.

Exercise. Daily exercise is good and stimulating to the circulation, bowels, and metabolism generally, and fresh air is also necessary. Walking (in moderation) provides both these, but swimming, riding, tennis and all athletics should be stopped after the early months. Housework in moderation is not harmful.

Rest. In addition to plenty of sleep in a room with open windows, the mother should have a good rest every afternoon, if possible with the foot of the bed raised so that the legs are above body level. She may need much rest in the later months, especially if complications such as varicose veins are present.

Supervision. This is given by doctor and nurse at the antenatal clinic, or otherwise privately, and is kept up throughout the pregnancy. The urine is tested, especially for albumen, every fortnight, and later every week, and the blood pressure is taken frequently, since it may indicate the onset of toxæmia. The blood is tested in order to discover if the mother is rhesus negative. The mother is urged to see her doctor at the first sign of any abnormality, and the nurse will explain to her the signs that might occur.

Attitude of Mind. It is to be hoped that the advent of the baby is looked forward to with joy. It is very important that the mother should feed her baby, even at the cost of sacrificing for a time her social pleasures, and she should be encouraged to regard it as her duty. A happy outlook is a great help, and is to be found often in the poorest surroundings, without the helpful conditions of pleasant rooms, leisure and comfort.

The Midwife.

Midwifery is a very vital section of the Health Service, and the profession has been the subject of several Acts of Parliament from 1902 onwards. By these Acts the professional status of the midwife has been made clear and her training and qualifications have been specified. To become a midwife, a State Registered Nurse must do one year's special training, and those who are not state registered must do two years. The two examinations of the Central Midwives' Board must be passed by the candidate, who then becomes a State Certified Midwife, and may use the letters S.C.M.

The midwife attends antenatal clinics, where she meets expectant mothers and learns to know them. Midwives who practise under the **Domiciliary Midwifery Service** work under the supervision of an officer, *The Non-Medical Supervisor of Midwives*, who is herself a senior qualified midwife. She is responsible to the Medical Officer of Health for the work of the service in his area. The midwife is responsible for the delivery in all normal births, sending for the doctor only in emergency. She visits the mother and baby for the next fourteen days and, in case of need, she can call upon the doctor, and through him the whole range of the health services.

At the end of the fortnight the health visitor takes over the care of the mother and baby.

A Maternity Nurse is one who has six months' training and then takes the first examination only. She works under the supervision of a doctor. She visits the expectant mother at intervals, and stays in the house when the baby is due. The doctor undertakes the delivery and, after the birth, the nurse has the care of mother and baby.

The Health Visitor

Health Visitors hold a unique position in the Health Service scheme, since they are concerned with the lives of the people from the cradle (and before) to the grave, with special responsibilities from prenatal months to five years of age. The health visitor needs to have great enthusiasm for her work, plenty of energy, and above all unlimited tact.

She must qualify for her post as follows:

(*a*) She must be a State Registered Nurse.

(*b*) She must be a State Certified Midwife if she wishes to take the combined health visitor/district nurse training; otherwise she must hold the certificate of Part I. of the Central Midwives' Board Examination.

(*c*) She must then qualify for the Health Visitor's Certificate of the Royal Sanitary Institute.

To gain this she takes a special course of nine months in a recognized centre, during which time she attends lectures and clinics and visits institutions that function under the Health Service. She also goes with a qualified health visitor making visits in the homes of the people. This practical experience is of the greatest value in her training.

When qualified, and holding an appointment, she is responsible to the Medical Officer of Health to whom her reports are made. Her duties include:

(1) Attendance at antenatal clinics, where she shares with the midwife the care of expectant mothers.

(2) Continued care of mothers at postnatal clinics.

(3) Care of the baby after the first two weeks, when she takes over from the midwife.

(4) Care of children up to five years.

(5) Care of women after stillbirths.

(6) Supervision of school-age children.

(7) Helping the aged.

(8) Supervision of tuberculous patients cared for in their homes.

(9) Giving advice and help on social problems when needed.

At all times, whether in clinics or in the homes, the health visitor both by advice and demonstration is *teaching health*. She has opportunities not shared by any other members of the health service team, of coming into close contact with the family in the home, and of observing their daily lives and their environment. She knows the wide range of services available under the Health Service Act, and when she meets with difficulties, and with cases where help is needed, she reports these to the Medical Officer of Health who then investigates and deals with the circumstances.

The Care of the Mother and New-born Baby.

The health visitor will have met the expectant mother at the antenatal clinic where she will have shared with the midwife the work of helping and advising her during her pregnancy. After the birth of the baby, either in hospital or in the home, the midwife takes charge for the first two weeks. At the third week the health visitor takes over until the child is five years old.

During the **first month** visits are made frequently, and the first visit, when she sees the mother in her own home environment, is of great interest to the health visitor. It is important to make sure that the mother is doing well, and that she is contented and happy to have the baby. If she is worried about the work and the family it may be possible to obtain a home help for her for a time. The health visitor enquires the baby's weight, observes its general appearance and its clothing, and discusses the feeding, giving any advice she thinks necessary and making sure that cod-liver oil and orange juice are given daily.

She is interested to know about the family—the father's occupation, the other children, if any, the sleeping arrangements and general cleanliness, and receives an overall idea of the family in its environment. She explains to the mother the importance of attending the clinics, and gives her the times.

The criterion of her success with the family is the extent to which she can gain the trust and confidence of the mother, who should feel that she has a friend who will always be ready to advise and help her. The most essential attribute for this success is tact.

Care during the First Year.

There will be much care and guidance needed as the baby grows and develops, and the mother is asked to bring the infant regularly to the Infant Welfare Clinic. In the early months feeding is of first importance, especially if the child is not breast fed, and later, between 4 and 5 months, the health visitor gives advice about weaning and mixed feeding and the diet that follows. When visiting the home she takes note of the baby's clothing and his cot.

Teething should not be troublesome in a normal infant, but convulsions sometimes occur if the nervous system is not very stable. In the case of a fretful baby it may be that the health visitor will need to explain to the mother that her way of handling him, and speaking to him might be the cause of his unrest, producing in him a sense of insecurity. The health visitor will consider whether the mother's failure to manage her baby happily may not be due to her own ill health, in which case attendance at the postnatal clinic may be the means of bringing her the help she needs.

During the later months of the first year the baby will begin to crawl and stand, and the health visitor will make sure that no harm can come to him. Fireguards are essential, and a strong baby can easily fall out of his pram if he is insecurely fastened in.

The mother will need advice concerning restful sleep, training in good habits, and daily routine.

Vaccination. This is usually arranged when the child is 3 or 4 months old. The parents' consent is obtained, often with difficulty, and they are asked to bring the infant to the clinic at a given time. If they neglect to do so the health visitor must do her best to persuade them.

Immunization against diphtheria. The need for this is urged in a letter to the parents when the child is about 10 months old. If they fail to bring him to the clinic it is the health visitor who will visit them and explain the great risk to their child of refusing to allow him to be immunized.

The Infant Welfare Clinic.

Clinics are established in convenient central positions, often near an infant school, and generally in adapted buildings. There is a pram shed near the entrance, and the mothers with their infants gather in a waiting-room in which are displayed a variety of show posters and flannelgraphs (previously made by health visitor students) which are a valuable method of health teaching. In the next room the infant is weighed and then inspected by the health visitor who proceeds to interview the mother. If it is a first postnatal visit, mother and baby pass on into the doctor's room where the infant is examined. Further examinations will be made at intervals, and it is here that the child will be vaccinated and immunized against diphtheria and whooping cough unless these procedures are carried out by the family doctor.

The mother may obtain a permit for an extra pint of milk daily for herself at a reduced price if the baby is breast fed. If the infant is artificially fed she can obtain National Dried Milk, full cream or half cream, as ordered by the doctor, at a reduced cost. She is also supplied with free cod-liver oil for the baby and with concentrated orange juice at a low cost.

All rooms at the clinic should be well warmed and well lighted and floor coverings should be washable and non-slip.

Care of Children from One to Five Years.

During the next two years, the health visitor will visit the home periodically, watching the growth and development of the child, and giving advice to the mother on his diet and care, including exercise, fresh air and clothing. She watches with interest his reaction to the home environment, his behaviour with other children and the development of his mind and intelligence.

The health visitor is present at the Child Welfare Clinics to which his mother brings him, and where he is seen at intervals by the doctor. At 5 years he is given a booster dose of diphtheria immunizing serum.

At 5 years he is due to start school, and theoretically will pass from the care of the health visitor to that of the school nurse, but often the health visitor is also the school nurse, in which case continuity of supervision is assured. In a final talk the mother may be glad to discuss the arrangements for his meals, his free morning milk, and the general school routine.

The Health Visitor and the School Child.

Since in country districts, the school nurse is frequently also the health visitor, her responsibilities with regard to school-age children are described in the section on "The School Child".

Other Duties of the Health Visitor

Care of the Aged and Infirm.

The health visitor is responsible for giving advice and help when necessary to old people who live alone, and are perhaps unable, through infirmity or illness, to keep themselves and their dwelling clean. Whenever she considers help is needed she reports the case to the Medical Officer of Health who, after investigation, may refer the matter to the Local Authority. Ultimately the case is put into the hands of a *Welfare Committee* set up by the Local Authority, and arrangements may be made for the aged person to be received into a home or a hospital.

Care of Premature Babies at Home.

Special care and attention is given to these babies by the midwife, and the health visitor follows up with extra visits, making sure that both mother and baby progress satisfactorily.

Visiting of Deprived and Foster Children and of Nurseries.

These visits and reports are the responsibility of the Children's Officer, but the children are also visited by the Health Visitor (see p. 256).

The Family in the Home

The health visitor will quickly gain an overall picture of the family and the home by her own observation and by information which she will gather with the greatest tact. She will come to know how many rooms the family occupies, if there is overcrowding, how the sleeping is arranged, if the rooms are clean and fresh, or the reverse. She will gain the confidence of the family who will soon welcome her visits. The ultimate reward of the health visitor for all her training and effort comes when she is received as a trusted friend in the homes she visits. No career is more satisfying nor has a wider scope. She sees the family against the background of the home, and the physical and mental well-being of each member is her personal concern. She is often asked for her advice and help in family difficulties, and she has all the resources of the Social Services to call upon. Even in a united family, where there is a happy atmosphere, circumstances may arise in which she can suggest and assist, while in unhappy homes there may be grave problems which she will report to the Medical Officer of Health. The health visitor of today is becoming more and more concerned with maintaining mental health of the family as a unit, and much of her training and subsequent experience is devoted to efforts to help the "problem families". When the fate of children is involved in the breaking up of a home, the Children's Officer deals with the matter, and he is able, under the provisions of the Children Act, to arrange for them to be received by adoption, or as "foster children" into a home where they will lead a normal life. Foster children remain under the supervision of the Local Authority, being visited at intervals by the health visitor until they are 18 years of age.

The Health Visitor and Infectious Diseases.

The health visitor plays an important part in the prevention and control of infectious diseases.

When a case has been notified to the Minister of Health she visits the home and, if the patient has been removed to hospital, she keeps a watch on the contacts.

If the patient is to be nursed at home she advises the parents or relatives concerning the precautions they should take with regard to the family, how to deal with fomites to prevent further spread of infection, and how best to manage the care of the patient. She keeps the contacts under observation and makes reports to the Minister of Health.

The health visitor has special responsibilities with regard to **diphtheria** and **pertussis,** she must persuade the parents to bring their children for immunization, and explain to them the danger of refusing to comply. During an outbreak of **smallpox** the health visitor helps with the campaign for vaccination, and assists with the visiting of contacts.

In the Health Service scheme for fighting **tuberculosis** the health visitor is a member of a team of specialists. She cannot undertake tuberculosis visiting unless she has received special training, and this, in many rural areas, is essential since the two branches of work are combined.

Many local authorities need full-time tuberculosis visitors who must be specially qualified.

The Tuberculosis Visitor is a State Registered Nurse who holds the certificate of the British Tuberculosis Association, and often also the Health Visitor's Certificate. Her duties consist of (a) work in the chest clinics, and (b) home-visiting.

(a) *In the chest clinics* the tuberculosis visitor sees all the patients and contacts who attend, and hears from the chest physician what instructions he has given each one with regard to diet, rest, etc. When she visits the patient in his home she is able to judge how far he is carrying out the doctor's orders. She can also give the physician useful reports about the patient's home conditions.

She is responsible in the clinics for applying and reading the tuberculin jelly tests, and giving intradermal injections for the Mantoux Test. She is also present at the B.C.G. vaccination sessions.

(b) *Home visiting* is of primary importance. Patients who have been newly notified need special consideration, care, and supervision. The health visitor must make sure that the patient and all members of the family understand the ways by which infection is conveyed and the means they must take in order to avoid spreading it.

This is health teaching of first importance. She will be concerned with the reactions of the family and may be able to help with her advice in readjustment of the home life.

She must try to persuade all *contacts* to attend the chest clinic for investigation, and must not desist until they have done so. The tuberculosis visitor pays follow-up visits to patients who have been discharged from sanatoria, and others who are allowed to work. She will inform the chest physician if home conditions do not appear to be satisfactory either from a material or psychological point of view, and all the resources of the Social Service will be made available as may be necessary. In these ways she shares, together with all the other members of the team, in the difficult work of the rehabilitation of the tuberculous patient.

Home Nursing Service

The District Nurse.

The nursing care of people in their own homes is a most valuable service in the Public Health scheme. For over 50 years the Queen's Institute of District Nurses, which is a voluntary organization, has undertaken the training of nurses for this service, and when in 1948 the National Health Service Act was passed, thousands of Queen's Nurses were working in all parts of the country. By the terms of the Act "Home

Nursing" became the responsibility of the Local Authorities, and the highly organized body of Queen's Nurses was available to them for the Home Nursing Service.

Queen's Nurses may be male or female, and all are State Registered. They are given special training in district nursing, including lectures, experience of practical work in the homes of the patients, visits to clinics, etc. The course is for six months, unless the nurse is a State Registered Midwife, or holds the Health Visitor's certificate, in which case she takes a four months' course.

At the end she sits an examination, and after passing she obtains a certificate and her name is entered on the Roll of Queen's Nurses.

The Queen's Institute also accepts nurses for combined training. With district nursing they may combine health visiting. The extra training gives the nurse a much wider choice of work. If her appointment is in a town she will probably do home nursing only, as there will be others specializing as midwives and health visitors. If she prefers the country she will probably be the midwife as well as the district nurse, and in the more underpopulated areas she is often the health visitor as well. This combined arrangement makes the district nurse's work much more interesting and satisfying. The nurse works under the direction of the patient's doctor, and has behind her, as do other public health personnel, all the help and resources of the service. Not all her patients are chronic cases; many are acutely ill, and the home nurses do a great service in relieving the pressure on hospital beds. There is, too, special interest in looking after patients in their homes, which is often more satisfying than caring for them in hospital beds away from their own environments.

There are many ways in which the district nurse can make use of the social services to help her patients:

she can procure for them the free loan of sick-room equipment, which otherwise they could not afford, or she may put them in the way of obtaining a "home help" to ease the difficulty of running the home while there is illness in the house.

Supervision of the work of district nurses is carried out by superintendents who pay occasional visits to their cases, give advice when needed, and send in reports of the work done. Many district nurses are glad to attend the refresher courses which are arranged for them at the Institute, the Royal College of Nursing and other centres.

The Home Help.

The Home Help Service has proved invaluable in many a time of household crisis. Domestic help is often needed in homes where there are ill or old people, or where a new baby is due to arrive, whether the mother is remaining at home or going to hospital.

This valuable service is part of the Local Government Health Service and Local Authorities appoint Home Help Organisers who run it. The work of the helps is supervised and homes are visited from headquarters. A charge is made, which varies with the circumstances. There is an Institute of Home Help Organisers, the members of which arrange schemes for the training of those who wish to take up this work.

The Almoner

In a large hospital there will be a Chief Almoner with a number of assistant almoners and an appropriate clerical staff.

The almoner's work is very exacting and far-reaching. The aim is to give help, in the best way available, to all patients who need it. To do this the almoner must not only understand the patient's needs, but she must have a complete knowledge of all the social services. She acts as a liaison officer between—on the one hand the hospital services with medical, surgical, nursing and ancillary staffs, and on the other hand the social services provided by local authorities, voluntary societies, and various rehabilitation schemes functioning under the Ministry of Labour.

The almoner is one of a team working for the welfare of the patient, and she acts in co-operation with the hospital staff, health visitors, district nurses, industrial staff in factories and other social workers.

Much of an almoner's work is concerned with helping patients to overcome difficulties and worries which hinder recovery. If the troubles are connected with the home, the health visitor may be able to help. When a patient is to be discharged it may be necessary to find a suitable convalescent home, or perhaps to arrange that the district nurse will visit him for further treatment. A patient with some permanent disablement may need help in readjusting his life and taking training for a different occupation. It is often necessary for an almoner to know something of a patient's social background to understand his difficulties and to help him in the way he needs.

In addition to this wide variety of work the almoner has the duty of teaching social medicine. She trains almoner students and gives lectures to medical students, nurses and social science students. The qualification needed for the position of almoner is the certificate of the Institute of Almoners, the course for which takes three years.

The Citizens' Advice Bureau

The Citizens' Advice Bureau is staffed by voluntary workers but receives a grant from the Local Authority. It exists to give information to individuals on any subject that presents difficulties. Details concerning legislation, pensions, regulations, welfare services, etc., are explained to all who apply.

SOCIAL MEDICINE AND INSURANCE

The present may be said to be the great age of social measures, several important Acts having been passed by Parliament within the last few years which, when in action, will greatly modify the social conditions of the people. These changes are not, however, entirely new—they date back from the seventeenth century and the new Acts replace the Poor Relief Act of 1601. Workmen's Compensation dates from 1907, though it was then limited to a few specially dangerous occupations. The National Health Insurance Act was introduced in 1911 as an insurance against loss by ill-health. The Unemployment Insurance Act of 1920 was limited to manual workers and non-manual workers earning not more than £250 a year. Old Age Pensions (non-contributory) were introduced in 1908, contributory pensions in 1925.

Beveridge Report. Lord Beveridge (then Sir William Beveridge) published his Social Insurance report in 1944 and the following Acts resulted:

1. *National Insurance (Industrial Injuries) Act, 1946,* which deals with workmen's compensation.

2. *The National Health Service Act, 1946,* which provides a comprehensive Health Service organized as shown on pp. 217, 218.

3. *The National Assistance Act, 1948,* which creates social services to provide for residential accommodation for the aged and infirm; arrangements for the welfare of the blind, deaf, and dumb; provision of temporary accommodation for those in urgent need—as through fire, flooding or eviction; and provision of aid to those whose needs are not met by National Insurance.

4. *Family Allowances and National Insurance Acts, 1945-1957.* These acts provide for:

(*a*) A payment of 8/- per week for the second child and 10/- each for the third and subsequent children.

(b) A unified and comprehensive scheme of National Insurance, based on the fact that practically everyone between school leaving age and pensionable age is an insured person. Three classes of persons are recognized according to employment status—employed, self-employed, and non-employed. Administration is through the Ministry of National Insurance with Regional and Local Offices working in close association with the Ministry of Labour.

TABLE OF RATES OF CONTRIBUTION, FEBRUARY 1958

Description of Contributor	Rates of Contribution for:			
	Employee	Employer	Self-employed	Non-employed
Men— Age 18 or over	9/5	8/1	11/6	9/1
Women— Age 18 or over	7/8	6/7	9/8	7/3
Boys— Under 18 ..	5/3	4/9	6/7	5/3
Girls under 18 ..	4/6	3/10	5/9	4/4

BENEFITS AND GRANTS

SICKNESS BENEFIT [*from* 6th February, 1958]

Men, single women and widows, aged 18 and over	50s. 0d.
Married women aged 18 and over	34s. 0d.
Boys and girls under 18	28s. 6d.

Additions for Dependants

One dependent adult	30s. 0d.
First or only dependent child	15s. 0d.
(Addition for each child after the first) ..	7s. 6d.

UNEMPLOYMENT BENEFIT [*from* 6th February, 1958]

Men, single women and widows, aged 18 and over	50s. 0d.
Married women aged 18 and over	34s. 0d.
Boys and girls under 18	28s. 6d.

Additions for Dependants

One dependent adult	30s. 0d.
First or only dependent child	15s. 0d.
(Addition for each child after the first)	7s. 0d.

MATERNITY BENEFIT [*from* 7th February, 1958]

Maternity Grant (*single payment*) ..	£12 10s. 0d.
Home Confinement Grant (*single payment*)	£5 0s. 0d.
Maternity Allowance	50s. 0d.

Additions for Dependants
 (*payable with Maternity Allowance only*)

One dependent adult	30s. 0d.
First or only dependent child	15s. 0d.
Addition for each child after the first	7s. 0d.

WIDOW'S BENEFIT [*from the first pension pay-day after* 27th January, 1958]

Widow's Allowance (first 13 weeks of widowhood)	70s. 0d.
Addition for first or only dependent child ..	20s. 0d.
Addition for each other child	12s. 0d.
Widowed Mother's Allowance, including addition for first or only child)..	70s. 0d.
Addition for each other child	12s. 0d.
Widowed Mother's Personal Allowance ..	50s. 0d.
Widow's Pension	50s. 0d.

GUARDIAN'S ALLOWANCE [*from the first pension pay-day after* 27th January, 1958]

For each child	27s. 6d.

RETIREMENT PENSIONS [*from the first pension pay-day after* 27th January, 1958]

Man or woman insured in own right	50s. 0d.
Addition for dependent wife, or for woman having care of child, under 60	30s. 0d.
Addition for first or only dependent child ..	15s. 0d.
Addition for each child after the first ..	7s. 0d.
Married woman in right of her husband's insurance	30s. 0d.
Widow in right of her husband's insurance ..	50s. 0d.

DEATH GRANT [*from* 3rd February, 1958]

Man or woman aged 18 and over.. ..	£25 0s. 0d.
Grants are reduced for men over 65 and women over 60	
Children under 3 years old	£7 10s. 0d.
aged 3 to 5 years	£12 10s. 0d.
aged 6 to 17 years	£18 15s. 0d.

CHAPTER XIV

SOCIAL SERVICES (*Continued*)

CHILDREN AND THE MENTALLY DEFECTIVE CHARTER

The Children Act (1948). This is described as the Children's Charter. It provides for the case of **deprived children**—that is, those who are deprived of a normal home life. By the Act they are the responsibility of the Home Office, and are in the immediate care of the Children's Officer who is appointed by the Local Authority. These children come under three categories:

  (*a*) Adopted children.
  (*b*) Foster children.
  (*c*) Children sent to approved schools and remand homes.

Since the health of the children is the concern of the Health Department, there is co-operation between the two departments.

Adopted Children. Acts have been passed to regulate the procedure of adoption, and a register of all adopted children is kept. The National Adoption Society will help both those who wish to arrange for adoption and those who wish to adopt. The Society gives advice about legal procedures.

Foster Children. These are children placed by their parents in the care of a foster mother who is paid by the parents. The Children's Officer is in charge of such children, and there are very comprehensive regulations to be observed by the foster parents. The homes are visited and inspected at intervals, and every care is taken to ensure that the children are properly looked after, and that the foster mother takes care of their health and well-being.

Child Minders. There are persons who take into their own homes, and care for, children under five years. The arrangement may be for daily or weekly care; if the latter the children are returned to their parents at weekends. By the Children Act the minders must be registered. The health visitor visits every month, and she must satisfy herself that the minders are fit persons, that their homes are clean and suitable, and that the children are properly fed and cared for.

Approved Schools

Juvenile delinquency is a problem which seriously taxes the Social Services. The number of children brought before the courts each year increases steadily. Experience in Approved Schools shows that when boys are given some real *practical* interest, with much patient and understanding help, they often become keen and capable young men. This is an indictment of their home upbringing. If, in their early years, their parents had helped them to be interested in hobbies and sports, they would not find their recreation later in joining lawless street gangs.

A hundred years ago the first "reformatory" was founded and was followed by others, all organized by private people who were distressed by the poverty and misery in the industrial towns and spent their time and money in rescuing children who, ill-fed and unruly, haunted the streets and ultimately filled the prisons. "Industrial Schools" for younger children were next established, and eventually Acts were passed making all these schools the responsibility of the Home Office. By the Children Act (1908) the "Children's Branch" of the Home Office was set up and Inspectors were appointed to visit the schools and make helpful suggestions for development. Many new schools have been opened to cope with the greater number of children brought before the courts. Some schools are now run by Local Authorities and some by voluntary associations with a "Manager" in control. All are designated "Approved Schools", and come under the *Home Office Children's Branch*. They are run by an enthusiastic body of headmasters and headmistresses who place the welfare of the child first, and education as of secondary importance.

The children sent in have all some background of unhappiness—wretched homes, neglect, lack of security and sometimes of affection. They need an ordered life, good food and care and, above all, an outlet for their energies.

The schools are graded Junior, Intermediate and Senior for boys, and Junior and Senior for girls. The children enter singly and are assessed individually.

Throughout, actual education is subordinated to the welfare of each particular child.

In the **Boys' Junior School** practical work is placed first, and includes handicrafts, gardening, music, etc., and always the child's character and temperament are studied as well as his capabilities. Some boys are so dull as to be almost classed as mental defectives, in which case Inspectors from the Home Office will visit and give advice.

The **Boys' Intermediate School** concentrates on gardening, engineering, carpentering, etc., with one, two or three days a week spent in the classroom.

The **Boys' Senior School.** These older boys often have a difficult start but they achieve really wonderful results. They run farms, learn carpentering and building, etc., with the object of making them feel that they are doing *necessary* work, not just being taught things. Usually the most self-assertive difficult type of boy will lose his hostile attitude and become co-operative and happy.

Girls' Junior Schools send the children out to nearby primary schools, and the **Senior Schools** teach them housework, dressmaking, cookery and laundry work.

The *health* of the children is the responsibility of the Medical Inspector of the Home Office, who may need to consult the Psychiatrist, since most of the children are there as the result of some emotional disturbance. There is a school doctor and a matron with a nurse to assist her who is often State Registered.

The school doctor visits weekly, examines each child on admission and holds a medical inspection every three months. His reports go to the Home Office. There is a sick bay with nurse's quarters, isolation room and surgery. Every child is immunized against diphtheria.

On admission children are often undernourished and neglected, but with good food, sleep and exercise they soon improve.

The *mental health* of the child is of first importance, and education and training are conditioned by it. Occasionally, a child needs to be examined by the Medical Psychologist from the Home Office who may refer him to the Child Guidance Clinic. The teachers and other staff do wonderful work in helping the child to overcome his difficulties, and the Head is invariably an outstanding personality who often remains a friend to the boy through life.

The school premises vary in type. Some are adapted mansions, some the original buildings of the old industrial schools, reconditioned, and others are separate houses or cottages with central dining and common rooms. There are playing fields, swimming bath, gymnasium, a library (sometimes with a boy librarian) and plenty of tools and other equipment.

Clubs are encouraged. There may be a Dramatic Club, Young Farmers' Club, Exploring Club (with bicycles), a seaside camp, and facilities to join the local scout troop.

There are no locks and bars, but not many children run away. Instead of "punishments", some privilege, such as an expedition, is taken away.

Some schools have a "Boys' Council" and the head-master may often consult this on school policy. Every effort is made to make the boy realize that he must be trustworthy.

On leaving the Approved School the child remains under the care of the Manager until the age of 18 or 21 years. He is given an outfit and often a sum of money and the Manager finds him a job.

The Home Office appoints to each area a Welfare Officer who visits the boy in his home and does everything possible to help him and his family.

Approved Schools are not hampered by policies, schemes and restrictions, they are therefore free to give all their energies to the welfare of each individual child in the way that will best help him.

Child Guidance Clinics

These clinics are provided as part of the National Health Service to help both children and parents when there is some emotional maladjustment in the child's relationships. A parent, who is in despair over the child's aggressiveness, cruelty, delinquency or nervous manifestations of some kind, takes him on the advice of the School Medical Officer to the clinic. The typical Child Guidance Clinic is run on a team basis with (a) the Child Psychiatrist (a qualified doctor special-izing in mental disorders in children) as the head of the team. Also in the team are (b) the Educational Psycho-logist, who thoroughly investigates the child's mental, educational and intellectual state and, by means of a series of tests and interviews, attempts to assess his intelligence, his educational standard, his emotional state and his reaction to his environment along with any particular deleterious psychological factors which may appear to influence him; (c) the Psychiatric Social Worker investigates the home environment, the school environment and the other social factors, interviews the parents and reports on these matters to the team. (d) Play Therapists and Psychotherapists are trained to treat the child after the diagnosis and assessment of his condition. In many cases a little simple advice to the parent suffices; in others simple therapeutic measures with some play therapy may be necessary. In the more severe cases, however, the child may be required to leave his home and is then sent to a boarding school or hostel and attends a different school, while obtaining treatment at the school or hostel.

The Care of Mental Defectives

In the process of growth the mind develops just as the body does. In some it develops quickly and to a higher level than normal so that these children become prize winners, the bright boys and girls and the pride of their parents and teachers. In others, however, the mind develops slowly and never reaches the average state. These children are the dullards, the backward pupils and the despair of their parents and teachers. In a minority this dullness is of such a degree that they are classed as educationally subnormal, and they have to be educated at special schools where the tempo is slower, more practical than theoretical work is done, and they are trained slowly for the less skilled jobs. In a small minority this dullness is of such a degree that the children are considered as ineducable and are excluded from school. They are then usually classed as Mental Defectives.

Mental Defective Colonies are provided for children (and adults) who are socially unacceptable either for the sake of others or for their own sake. An attempt is made in these colonies to train them for life in the open market, and success is obtained with some, while others become able to earn their living provided they have some supervision.

Mental Disorders in Adults

All cases of severe mental disease are cared for in mental hospitals to which they are admitted on certification by doctors and by a magistrate's order. The procedure in these cases is regulated by the *Lunacy Acts*. In 1930 the *Mental Treatments Act* was passed, by which patients may ask to be admitted for treatment in mental hospitals. On recovery they may be discharged, returning again on their own initiative if necessary. They are known as *voluntary patients* and are not subject to the enactments of the Lunacy Laws.

CHAPTER XV

SOCIAL SERVICES (*Continued*)

SCHOOL AGE, OCCUPATIONAL HEALTH, OLD AGE

THE SCHOOLCHILD

FROM 3–5 years children go to Nursery Schools.

From 5–7 or 8 years they attend Infant Schools.

From 8–11 years they attend County Primary Schools.

At 11 years an examination is taken, and those who are most successful go to Grammar Schools. Of those who do not reach this standard some go to Modern Schools, and others to Technical Schools.

Grammar School. Children receive a thorough general education in all subjects. The work is intensified in the sixth form, and becomes more specialized as they study for different professions. The Certificate of Education may be taken at three levels; Ordinary Level, Advanced Level (2 or 3 subjects) and Scholarship Level.

Modern School. Children who pass into Modern Schools are of varying degrees of intelligence but usually have a practical bent. Some are backward or even sub-normal. They are given a good all-round education with special emphasis on practical subjects. Even the theoretical work is correlated and combined with practical experience. Much use is made of radios, films, art, handicrafts, etc., and the special interests of each child are studied.

Examinations are taken in which oral and practical

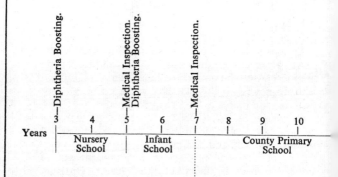

Supervision of Health Visitor.
Toddlers' Clinic.
Free Milk Daily.
Free Meals.

Supervision of School Nurse ......
Dental Clinic each Term.   ....
Cleanliness Inspection each Term...
Free Milk Daily. ....
Meals Service. ....
Physical Training at All Stages. ....

Diphtheria Boosting.

Medical Inspection.
Diphtheria Boosting.

Medical Inspection.

Years 3   4   5   6   7   8   9   10
          Nursery   Infant   County Primary
          School   School   School

COUNTY PRIMARY SCHOOL

FIG. 69.—THE CAR

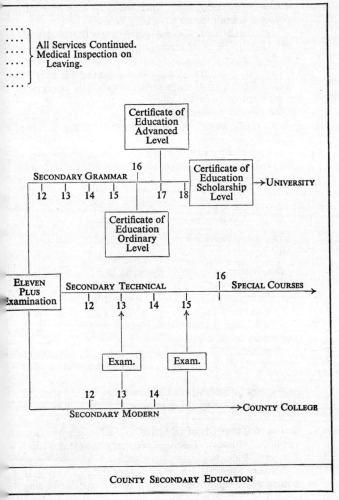

All Services Continued. Medical Inspection on Leaving.

Certificate of Education Advanced Level

16
SECONDARY GRAMMAR

12 13 14 15 17 18

Certificate of Education Scholarship Level →UNIVERSITY

Certificate of Education Ordinary Level

ELEVEN PLUS Examination

SECONDARY TECHNICAL

12 13 14 15

16 SPECIAL COURSES →

Exam. Exam.

12 13 14
SECONDARY MODERN

→COUNTY COLLEGE

COUNTY SECONDARY EDUCATION

THE SCHOOLCHILD.

results are stressed, after which the child may pass into technical school, or go to county college.

Technical School. General education is thorough and, in addition, the child receives special technical training in the subject chosen, *e.g.* industry, agriculture, commerce, art, pre-nursing, etc. When the child is over 16 years of age part-time general education is continued and advanced technical courses are given.

Residential Secondary Schools are contemplated in which there would be more opportunity for a fuller social life.

County Colleges are planned to provide further part-time education for those who need it after school-leaving age.

Nurseries and Nursery Schools

These are provided by Local Authorities and are of three types:

Day Nurseries where mothers can leave their children while they go out to work. Children of any age up to five years are taken. The mothers bring them after 7.30 a.m. and fetch them by 6.30 p.m. The Local Authority makes charges which may vary according to the family income.

Residential Nurseries where children stay for longer periods while the mothers are away in hospital or ill at home.

Nursery Schools where children from 3 to 5 years old attend from 9 a.m. to 3.30 p.m. during school term times.

The staff consists of a Matron and a Deputy Matron, qualified Nursery Teachers, Nursery Assistants and Nursery Students.

Nursery Students are girls who are taking a two-year course of training, spending two days a week attending a further education course, and the rest of the time in the nursery for practical work. At the end they take the examination for the certificate of the National Nursery Examination Board.

Nursery Assistants must have taken a short course in Child Care.

The Nursery

The Nursery must be a bright and happy place where the children will be cared for in pleasant surroundings by specially trained Nursery Nurses and Nursery Teachers.

The rooms must be light and airy and well-warmed and there should be a garden or plenty of playing space out-of-doors. The indoor decorations should be light, with bright, attractive curtains, etc., and chairs, tables and cupboards of a suitable height for the under-fives.

The members of the staff are concerned to make the children happy and confident and to give them that sense of security which is so vital in their early years. The child, feeling the sympathy and affection of the adults who are caring for him and training him, will develop as he would do in a happy home.

His training stresses daily ordered routine.

Toilet. He gradually learns to manage his own washing, dressing, etc., with special emphasis on keeping separate his own toilet articles.

Meals are so managed that meal-time is a happy un-hurried occasion. Sometimes meals are taken out-of-doors and, in any case, the service is orderly and every-thing clean and attractive. The diet for the midday meal is carefully balanced, containing milk, eggs and meat or fish to supply the protein that growing children need, and always vegetables and fresh fruit.

Rest. All the children have a daily rest time. Low stretcher beds are provided and each child has his own, suitable to his size, and his own blanket. They sleep on these out-of-doors in fine weather.

Play. Children at play show their individuality, observation and imagination. They should be provided with as many as possible of the materials they enjoy using; spades and pails, see-saws and swings, trees (if there are any), benches, bricks, sand and water are some of the out-of-door needs; and indoors, bricks, clay, paints, paper, picture books and any available toys.

Health. The staff of a nursery is responsible for the health and cleanliness of the children. Milk, cod-liver oil and orange juice are provided free. All precautions are taken against spread of infection, and any child who appears to be ill is isolated in a separate room until the doctor has seen him. In some nurseries immunization against diphtheria is carried out, and also against whooping cough.

Nurseries not run by Local Authorities are obliged under the Children Act to be registered and inspected. The health visitor visits every month, and her inspection includes the children's meals, their daily rest and the keeping of the register. Nurseries must be properly staffed and the children are under medical supervision. The health visitor has right of entry into the premises, and records are sent to the Local Authority.

Special Schools for Handicapped Pupils

The Blind. Infants up to five years who do not remain at home, are received in residential nursery schools which belong to the National Institute for the Blind. From five to sixteen years they receive primary education in special schools, and during these years any who show exceptional ability are transferred to a secondary school for the blind. At sixteen years they start to train for a chosen occupation. They may choose to be shorthand typists, machine-knitters, manual workers in various trades, or they may study for law, physiotherapy, music and other professions. Very gifted children may go to a University, working with the normal students, but using Braille textbooks.

Aged blind people are helped in various ways. Local Authorities provide a home visiting service. The visitor teaches them to read embossed type, teaches them crafts, sees that they receive the available extra financial help, and that, if poor, they are supplied with free wireless sets (for which the licences are paid). She tells them about the National Library for the Blind, and the "Talking Book"—a gramophone which plays recorded books.

The deaf are of two classes: (a) children who are born deaf and therefore have never heard speech; (b) adult deaf people, not all of whom are totally deaf.

(a) *Deaf children* attend special schools, many of which are run by voluntary societies. They are trained to lip-read and talk by sign language. At the same time they study the subjects in a normal syllabus according to their ages, and ultimately many are able to enter for recognized examinations.

(b) *The Adult Deaf.* There are many voluntary welfare societies to care for these people. They are trained in skilled crafts at which they are often very clever, but it is not always easy to place them where they can earn their living. Welfare workers for the deaf are trained and qualify by taking the examination of the Deaf Welfare Examination Board. The "partially-deaf" are helped by the welfare societies in many ways. There are clubs that they may join, where lip reading classes are arranged, and social activities are provided.

Physically handicapped children who suffer from some crippling defect are under the care of the School

9

Medical Officer who will arrange for their education in a suitable school or home.

" Disabled persons " who are ex-service patients are eligible for many benefits, and they, as well as other adults, are helped to train for some types of work that will give them interesting occupation and financial profit.

There are special schools where **subnormal children, epileptics, maladjusted children** and those who suffer from **speech defects** receive specialized education.

Delicate pupils who do not come under any of the above categories yet who are not strong enough to attend ordinary schools. Education of these children may be in boarding or day schools, and in every case they receive the same medical and dental care as that provided in normal schools, and free milk. The size of the classes is limited for each category and varies from to twenty or thirty. Many pupils over the age of sixteen are able to take courses of training while still continuing their general education, and are able ultimately to qualify for a profession or trade.

The School Health Service

The health of the school child is the responsibility of the School Medical Officer who is often the Medical Officer of Health. He has as his assistant a School Nurse.

Regular medical, dental and cleanliness inspections are carried out in all schools.

The hygiene of the classroom is important. Ventilation must be efficient, the ventilators being placed at ceiling level. At a lower level there must be windows that can be opened as required. Lighting should be adequate. The diffused type is best, and the lights should be so arranged as to avoid glare and shadows on desks and work tables.

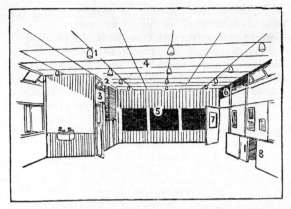

FIG. 70.—A MODERN SCHOOL-ROOM.

(1) Simple low-brightness light fittings; (2) Louvred blinds housed in ceiling; (3) Opening lights from sill to head level, with fixed pane over, and ventilator at ceiling level; (4) Sound-absorbing and light-reflecting ceiling panels; (5) Avoid a strong contrast of light and dark between the chalkboard and the background; (6) Blinds for dim-out purposes; (7) Door with glazed panel; (8) Cupboard forming working surface, with sliding doors down to the floor.

Reproduced from The New Secondary Education *by permission of the Controller of H.M. Stationery Office.*

School Meals. This subject is foremost in the scheme of the Board of Education. Free meals for all school children is the ultimate aim of their policy but at present there are not sufficient facilities for this and small charges are made in most cases. Certain classes of children, however, receive free meals—those whom the school doctor decides are insufficiently nourished to profit by the education and physical training received. Meals are served at school canteens or feeding centres. The calorie value is carefully calculated with regard to the age group in question, and the meal is balanced so that sufficient first-class proteins, calcium and vitamins are included. The cooking, serving and general behaviour are all under supervision. All children receive free milk (two-thirds of a pint daily).

Physical Training. Gymnasia, swimming baths and playing fields are essential in the education scheme. Physical training and organized games either in the gymnasium or out of doors develop in the child not only fitness of the body but also alertness of mind and a team spirit. Dancing and swimming have each a special value. Camping is a valuable experience (see p. 114) and holidays abroad for elder children are arranged by many schools.

The School Nurse

The school nurse must be State Registered and she often holds the Health Visitors' Certificate as well. The health visitor is frequently also the school nurse.

There are three **routine medical examinations** of the children:

    (1) When the child enters;

    (2) on leaving the primary school;

    (3) on leaving the secondary school.

Medical examinations include eye tests, dental inspection (this is done yearly) and general observation for any defects which may handicap the children and need treatment.

The school nurse is present at these inspections. The child's intelligence quotient is filled in by the teacher.

Cleanliness inspections are undertaken by the school nurse each term, convenient times having been arranged with the teachers.

These inspections are very thorough, and include:

    (*a*) The hair and scalp. If found to be verminous the child's home is visited, and the mother is given 24 hours to clean up the head using suleo which is given to her with instructions how to use it. If after this the head is still not clean the nurse does the treatment herself. If the mother persistently refuses to co-operate the child is sent home and the school enquiry officer is informed.

(*b*) The neck, ears, mouth and teeth are inspected.

(*c*) The finger nails are inspected for nail-biting.

(*d*) The way the child sits, stands, and walks will be observed.

(*e*) The clothing, and particularly the shoes are noted.

Any defects found during the examination are reported to the School Medical Officer, and home visits are made when necessary. Twice during school years— at about 5 and 9 years old—children who were immunized against diphtheria in infancy are given a booster dose of T.A.F. (Toxoid Antitoxin Floccules).

ENVIRONMENT

Whatever may be a child's inherited characteristics, the environment both physical and mental in which he grows and develops has a profound effect on his well-being and determines to a large extent the pattern of his behaviour.

Mental Environment. This is by far the more important. A child who is brought up in a home where there is tension and unhappiness will feel a sense of fear and insecurity which will have reactions on his mind and his physical health, affecting him throughout his life.

Physical Environment. This includes all the surroundings and conditions in which the child grows up and the adult lives and works. Housing, working premises, diet, clothing and fresh air are all part of the picture.

Social security is the foundation on which homes are built, and the primary need is for good and sufficient *housing*. A suitable number of rooms for the size of the family, sanitary services, warmth, sun and fresh air and playing ground for the children are some of the basic necessities for the home. Between this ideal housing target and the lowest category, listed as slums and due to be demolished, there are some millions of old houses in disrepair, each inhabited by a varying number of families. Overcrowding, basement dwellings, damp walls and leaking roofs are the constant preoccupation of sanitary inspectors. Such conditions, added to poverty and poor diet, provide among other adversities a suitable background for the spread of tuberculosis. For example the health visitor may discover a newly notified case of pulmonary tuberculosis sleeping in the same room as the children, and the combined efforts of the Health Service team and the Welfare Committee will be needed to find a solution of the problem.

The same conditions of overcrowding and poverty are a predisposing factor in the high incidence of *acute rheumatism* in childhood. This is the cause of thousands of deaths from heart disease in later life and, in most cases, the years between have been made difficult by ill health. Public health authorities are making great efforts to cope with this disease, and intensive research is proceeding. Rheumatism Supervisory Clinics have been set up in some big towns to keep in touch with schools and to keep a lookout for the "pre-rheumatic child", *i.e.* the weakly, ill-nourished type, that so often develops rheumatism.

It is found that if these children can be removed for some time to special schools in the country where they lead an open-air life with sunshine and good food, their resistance is improved and the disease averted. These are prophylactic measures.

Another problem arises connected with the children who do develop rheumatism. The heart is often badly damaged, and months of rest are necessary if they are to be saved from becoming lifelong "cardiac cripples". Special "heart hospitals", or wings of hospitals, are the best means of dealing with the difficulty, since the children are usually of the artisan class and their parents are not able to give the care needed. For six months or more they have rest, good food, fresh air and sunlight, education, and gradual retraining of the heart.

As the housing problem, despite its magnitude, is gradually solved, the standard of living should be correspondingly improved, and the full effects of the scheme of social welfare should be apparent.

Apart from a well built house of suitable size, provided with efficient Sanitary Services and a good water supply, it is essential that much thought should be given to the provision of **playgrounds for the children.**

The question of how and where the child is to spend his free time when he comes home from school is of the greatest importance. Young children need plenty of playing space and something they can use for constructing and experimenting in their own way. Neither streets nor concrete playgrounds are satisfactory for their needs, and often fields, trees and parks are too far away.

A recent development, which originated in Denmark and is now being tried in various towns in this country, is the "junk playground". Rough ground is chosen for the site, where digging is possible, and any kind of available material is provided: planks, tubs, an old door, a derelict car, bricks, sand, old sacks, etc. With these the children construct most ingenious caves, houses, ships and other wonders, and interested parents and friends often supply needed materials. A "leader" (a trained nursery school teacher is best) helps in their projects with advice, but never tries to order or organize. The children must feel free and responsible.

The child's indoor activities are usually hampered in his home environment by lack of space and of any spot that he can call his own. He should be given some place —a cupboard, a shelf or even a large box where he can keep his treasures.

When children reach the secondary school age there is much more opportunity for constructive use of leisure. School clubs, libraries, sports and other social activities give them a wide choice of interests. Each of these recreations has its own advantages and there is no need for a child's interests to be bounded by his home environment. A camping holiday widens his outlook, as well as providing opportunity for enjoyment and training, and if he is fortunate enough to be one of a holiday party abroad he will have a rich experience. Even if these good things do not come his way, he can often find absorbing interest in a library, making use of maps and pictures and constructing his own models. All large schools should be provided with libraries and reading rooms for the children's use, and whatever bias they show towards any particular subject or activity should receive every encouragement.

OCCUPATIONAL HEALTH

The health and working conditions of between twenty and twenty-five million workers are now rigorously controlled by the terms of the **Factory Acts** of 1937 and 1948, under the administration of the Ministry of Labour and National Service. These Acts are the culmination of successive efforts to improve by legislation the lot of the workers who in the early part of the nineteenth century were herded together in badly lit, ill-ventilated buildings to work through their twelve-hour day. Important milestones on the road were the appointment of Factory Inspectors and later of Medical Inspectors. By the Act of 1937 fourteen industrial diseases were made notifiable, and rules were laid down for the safety and welfare of workers. The 1948 Act added to these rules and designated the qualified doctor appointed by the Chief Inspector of Factories as the "Factory Doctor". New Regulations are added from time to time dealing with special precautions and other details.

The Industrial Injuries Act (1948) deals with compensation payable for accidents and with pension allowances for permanent disablement.

The Works Medical Officer is concerned with maintaining the health of the worker and with supervising their working environment.

He must understand the processes that are carried on, and he should have direct contact with the management so that he may advise on matters affecting the health of the worker.

He supervises the First Aid Services and sees that his staff is instructed in any special treatment that is likely to be needed, such as artificial respiration where there is risk of carbon monoxide poisoning. He makes any necessary medical examination of workers who are employed in processes that entail special health risks, such as tar epithelioma.

With regard to the fitness of workers returning after sickness the Works Medical Officer collaborates with the Medical Practitioner and the Welfare Authorities.

The Occupational Health Nurse is a State-registered nurse who has taken a public health training and/or a course in Industrial Nursing. She is responsible to the Medical Officer, and may have one or more partly trained assistants.

She has charge of the surgery where she does any daily dressings, and treatments to minor injuries and ailments.

She assists the doctor at examinations of employees, and through her daily contact with them she may be

able to give useful help. She has the very important
duty of looking after the first aid equipment both in the
ambulance room and throughout the works.

The **Factory Inspector** is responsible for the safety of
machinery and the general welfare arrangements.

The **Sanitary Inspector** does regular inspections and
reports are made to the Local Authority.

General Factors that Affect the Health of the Worker

1. **Temperature.** Workrooms must be comfortably
warm, but the cooling power of the air must be maintained so that the physiological heat regulation mechanism of the workers may function. There must be moving
currents of air to prevent excessive heat or moisture.

2. **Ventilation.** This is secured by moving currents of
air and is vitally important. The most modern method
of achieving good ventilation is by means of ducts
running high up along the walls with powerful suction
fans some of which extract air while others draw in
fresh air. Duct openings are spaced at intervals.
Where dust, fumes or gases are produced special
exhaust ventilators are fixed.

3. **Lighting.** There must be good lighting in work-
rooms but without glare, and above all without casting
shadows. Local lights may be needed over work
benches. Bad lighting causes eye strain and accidents.

4. **Overcrowding.** This is forbidden by law.

5. **General Cleanliness.** The general condition and
cleanliness of premises with regard to walls, floors and
ceilings is prescribed by law.

Welfare

1. **Sanitary Arrangements.** Lavatory accommodation
must be sufficient; an ample number of wash-basins
must be provided with soap, nail-brushes and towels or

air-driers. Often baths, both plunge and shower, are supplied. Each worker has his own locker and cupboard, and there are facilities for drying clothes.

2. **Seats.** Where there are opportunities for workers to sit at their work seats of suitable height must be provided.

3. **Water.** There must be an ample supply of drinking water with an upward jet for drinking in preference to drinking vessels.

4. **The Canteen.** This is a most important part of the facilities in factories. Good meals of high calorie value at low cost are provided in pleasant surroundings. A Catering Officer is in control and is responsible for supervising the cleanliness of the kitchens, dining-rooms, etc.

Inspection. H.M. Inspectors may inspect every part of a factory as may also Officers of the Local Authority as far as their duties require.

Occupational health is concerned with:

    (*a*) Industrial Diseases.

    (*b*) Accidents.

Industrial Diseases

Many of these are notifiable. They may be classified as follows:

Diseases Due to Inhalation of Fumes or Dust.

Poisoning with Fumes. Most of these cases occur among workers who work with *industrial solvents* such as *benzene, carbon tetrachloride, carbon bisulphide*, and some of the *alcohols*. They are used in various processes, *e.g.*, as rubber solvents; in cellulose spraying, lacquers and varnishes; in the manufacture of artificial silk and leather; in oil extraction from seeds, nuts and bones; and in fire extinguishers. Some of them are inflammable.

Prevention of Poisoning by Fumes. Every possible

precaution is taken to prevent fumes escaping into the air, to be inhaled by the workers:

1. Exhaust ventilators are fixed at points where fumes are produced.

2. General ventilation of the work-rooms is ensured by extraction fans.

3. Sometimes the process which evolves the fumes can be enclosed in an air-tight cabinet.

4. In some cases the workers wear respirators, and these may have long tubes supplying them with air.

5. Medical examinations of the workers take place at frequent intervals.

6. Special precautions against fire are taken if the solvents used are inflammable.

Carbon monoxide fumes may occasionally overcome workers in blast furnaces, and gas-welders may be affected by these fumes.

"Dust" Diseases. These are caused by inhaling irritant dusts in certain occupations.

Silicosis is fibrosis of the lungs caused by inhaling fine particles of flint (silica). Asbestos workers are specially liable to develop it, also grinders, stone-masons, pottery workers and workers making scouring powders. Colliers are liable to a chronic lung disease—pneumokoniosis—and cotton-spinners also develop lung disease.

Poisonous dusts, such as arsenic used in making paints and sheep dip, and in preserving skins; manganese used in the manufacture of batteries for torches and electric bells; mercury used by furriers and in making thermometers; and T.N.T. used in explosives.

Symptoms of these vary and are very severe.

Allergic dusts, for example chromic acid, causing asthma, catarrh or urticaria.

Infectious Dusts. The chief infections produced by

these is anthrax, a disease of cattle caused by a sporing bacillus. Workers who handle hides and wool may inhale the spores in dust and develop lung disease, or the skin may be infected through an abrasion.

Prevention. This is mainly achieved by the substitution, when possible, of harmless substances, as is done in the manufacture of china.

All means are used to keep the air as dust free as possible; ventilation systems must be efficient; hooded exhaust fans are fitted over work tables; masks may be worn; moist methods are used when possible; cleaning of floors, benches, tables, etc., where dust may lodge is very important.

Electric Arc Welding.

This requires special mention since so much welding is done now on machinery and all kinds of metal constructions. Welders are subject to many risks—inhaling fumes, electric shock, burns, damage to the eyes from rays, and general ill health. Measures for their protection include the provision of masks and air tubes.

Apart from special protective measures, there should be ample washing facilities, protective clothing changed frequently, care that the position of workers is easy, good lighting, supervised canteens where well balanced meals are served, and regular medical supervision.

Industrial Dermatitis.

This is the commonest of the industrial diseases. Some of the chief causes are: petroleum oils; solvents, *e.g.* chrome and other acids; alkalis, *e.g.* lime; dyes, paints and many other chemical substances. Coal tar and mineral oils may cause warts which may become malignant.

Preventive measures include supplying protective clothing for workers, providing good washing facilities, and seeing that anti-dermatitis soap and barrier creams are used on the arms and parts liable to be splashed.

Accidents

Everything possible is done to reduce the number of industrial accidents. Inexperienced and younger workers are trained and supervised and the Safety Officer or Works Manager is responsible for seeing that the safety regulations are carried out. There are many minor accidents in various industries and a small number of serious ones. Accidents must be reported to the District Inspector if there is loss of life, or if the worker is disabled for more than three days.

Accidents are usually caused by machinery not properly guarded; by workmen falling from heights, scaffolding, etc.; through being hit by a heavy object falling from above, or by careless handling of tools. Contributory causes are: (1) Fatigue: working on long shifts and going too long without food: the mental and physical reactions are slowed down and serious accidents may occur. (2) Bad conditions of environment: poor lighting; insufficient ventilation; overcrowding. One of the most important regulations enforces guarding of machinery. All dangerous machinery and moving parts must be fenced off. Other regulations concern steam boilers, electrical apparatus, cranes, inflammable substances, etc.

The factory nurse attends to daily treatment of minor injuries and assists the doctor when necessary. She also has the care of the first aid boxes which must always be ready for instant use.

Rehabilitation

One of the outstanding developments since the last war has been the fillip given to the measures of rehabilitation. The aim of rehabilitation is very simply put as the attempt to get the patient back into the best possible condition, mentally and physically, in the shortest possible time. All too often in the past, and indeed too often in the present, the patient having received his treatment at the hands of the general practitioner or the hospital is then allowed to drift back, not returning to his work, or told to go easily which he proceeds to do for the rest of his life. In most of the modern-minded hospitals, the patient is assessed early, and his subsequent treatment is directed to qualify him in all ways to return to his previous job. Sometimes this is not easy. It may be that he is unable to do so on account of some permanent disability. In such cases a conference is held between the Consultant concerned, the Almoner and the Disablement Resettlement Officer (D.R.O.) of the Ministry of Labour, and an attempt is made to fit the patient into a job within his ability and to his liking. In some cases this will require special training or a sheltered type of occupation for some months or years. For such purposes the Ministry of Labour has set up Training Centres and Sheltered Workshops, *e.g.* Remploy Factories. Too much stress should not, however, be placed on these special measures. The majority of patients who require re-habilitation, require it because they have lost confidence in themselves and the purpose of rehabilitation in these cases is to return their confidence to them, usually by gradually increasing their work and showing them how much they can do by themselves.

CARE OF THE AGED

The welfare of old people is a matter that requires constant consideration. In the past they were cared for by their own families, and those with no means or families were looked after in residential homes run by a wide variety of religious societies, and a number of small "almhouses" provided by trusts. The residue were received in "institutions". In 1908 old age pensions were introduced and in 1925 they were made contributory. If the amount of the pension is not sufficient to keep them under changed economic conditions, the old people may apply to the National Assistance Board for extra help.

In 1940 the National Old People's Welfare Committee was set up by the National Council of Social Service to co-operate with the existing voluntary societies (which now include many organizations), in the work of caring for the aged by providing help for them in a variety of ways.

Old people's clubs are established; visitors call on those who are lonely; "meals on wheels" services are provided and domestic help is sometimes arranged. Every year sees more residential homes opened and the provision of many more is contemplated.

Under the National Assistance Act Local Authorities have the duty of providing these homes but much of the work is done by voluntary organizations helped by grants obtained from various sources by the Old People's Welfare Committee.

Residential homes are so greatly needed that, in some cases, the authorities have of necessity made use of the premises of old "institutions". The old people in them are called "residents" (not "inmates") and are allowed a certain amount of liberty, some personal possessions, and their own clothes. The buildings are improved to provide more comfort.

A notable advance has been made by some Local Authorities who, realizing that old people differ widely in type, have opened smaller homes, comfortable and free from restrictions.

Nevertheless, by far the greater number of retirement pensioners and other old people of limited means do not wish to give up their independence and live in communal homes, however thoughtfully organized. It seems that simple one-room flatlets at a low rental and with a communal dining-room would be a happy solution for many. Quite different is the case of *the aged sick and infirm people* who live alone and are not able to look after themselves. By a provision in the Public Health Act power is given to the Medical Officer of Health to order removal of such old people to a hospital or suitable home.

CHAPTER XVI

PREVENTION AND CONTROL OF INFECTIOUS DISEASES

METHODS by which the spread of infectious diseases is controlled include:

(a) Notification.

(b) Isolation of the patient, usually in hospital.

(c) Disinfection of fomites and sometimes of premises.

(d) Search for the source of infection, which in some cases includes carriers.

(e) Observation of contacts.

(f) Vaccination and immunization against diphtheria, tuberculosis and whooping cough.

(g) Teaching by health visitors and others and by means of posters, etc.

The responsibility for the prevention of spread of an infectious disease rests with the Medical Officer of Health and he is assisted by Sanitary Inspectors and Health Visitors.

Notification. All cases of notifiable diseases (see p. 128) are notified by the general practitioner to the Medical Officer of Health who reports them to the Ministry of Health.

Isolation of the Patient. This varies with the disease. Smallpox cases go to a special smallpox hospital, and other infectious diseases to an infectious diseases hospital or to special wards in a general hospital. Children who go to boarding schools are nursed in the sanatorium there, and some diseases, *e.g.* measles, are nursed in the homes.

Disinfection. The articles that need care in handling and disposal vary in different types of infection and are indicated on pp. 288–293.

Room disinfection is not normally carried out, but special measures are taken in premises where a smallpox patient has lived and worked.

Search for the Source of Infection. The method of search varies with the disease. In cases of *intestinal infections*, such as enteric fever, the search is often prolonged. The water supply is examined, the sewage disposal arrangements investigated, specimens of milk are tested in the laboratory and, if necessary, search may have to be made for a carrier either among milkers or those who handle food.

If the infection is *infantile gastro-enteritis*, the babies' cot linen, squares, bottles and teats, milk, towels and toilet articles, may be responsible for the spread of infection conveyed by hands or flies.

Diphtheria may be spread by droplet infection from a carrier who will be discovered when swabs are taken.

In cases of *puerperal sepsis* and *scarlet fever* nose and throat swabs may reveal a carrier of hæmolytic streptococci. In cases of *lung tuberculosis* mass radiography of contacts may reveal the unnotified case.

Observation of Contacts. This is always important but especially in the event of a case of smallpox. As soon as the diagnosis is made and the patient removed to a smallpox hospital all known contacts are vaccinated and visited daily. The search for contacts is carried into every place the patient has visited, and centres are set up where people living in the area are urged to attend for vaccination. The patient's home and the premises in which he has worked receive a thorough disinfection and cleaning, and the same applies to any public vehicle he is known to have used. Chickenpox is usually made notifiable for the time being.

Outbreaks of infectious diseases in schools are the

cause of much disruption of studies. Measles, scarlet fever, whooping cough, chickenpox and mumps are the common cause of epidemics. A child who develops the disease is sent home, and comes under the charge of the family doctor. The health visitor visits if the child remains at home and advises the parents about nursing care and how to prevent spread of infection. She keeps a watch on contacts and makes reports to the doctor if necessary.

VACCINATION AND IMMUNIZATION
Immunity

When pathogenic bacteria gain entrance to the body this is termed *infection*.

The body puts up a resistance by means of its defence mechanism and the result depends on (*a*) the state of its defences, (*b*) the general nutrition of the body, (*c*) the dose and virulence of the organisms.

The defences of the body are:

      (1) Leucocytes which ingest and destroy bacteria.

      (2) Antibodies which assist in the process.

Leucocytes.

These are swiftly mobilized to attack bacteria when they are present in the blood and tissues. Many invading bacteria produce powerful toxins which either kill leucocytes or so inhibit their action that the bacteria may get the upper hand.

Antibodies and **antitoxins.**

These are substances formed in the body (in the liver, spleen and lymphoid tissue), in response to the presence of bacteria. Special antibodies are produced for each type of organism. If they are already present in the blood stream the body is well equipped to resist the infection. Therefore every effort is made to ensure that the body is provided with the special antibodies against the bacteria that are most likely to invade it. The organisms that stimulate production of antibodies are " antigens ".

The Means by which the Body is Provided with Antibodies

(1) **Inherited Immunity.** The baby receives from his mother various antibodies present in her blood, and these give him protection for a time from those specific diseases.

(2) **Acquired Immunity.**

(a) *Active Immunity.* The specific antibodies to fight any infection can be produced in the body only by means of the presence of the particular organism concerned. There are three ways by which the special bacteria needed for the purpose can be introduced into the body:

(1) The individual may have an attack of the disease, in which case the bacteria are present in immense numbers and antibodies are produced in order to help in their destruction.

(2) He may constantly take in the bacteria in small doses by frequent contact with infection so that over a length of time his body builds up a store of the specific antibodies.

(3) He may be given injections of small doses of the bacteria which have been prepared and weakened in the laboratory by various processes. The preparation is a *vaccine*.

In these three ways the body may be stimulated to become active in producing antibodies, so the result is spoken of as **active immunity.** The duration of effectiveness varies for different diseases.

(b) *Passive Immunity.* In this case the patient is in a state of emergency. Either he is already suffering from the disease (*e.g.* a case of diphtheria), or it is feared that he may have been infected (*e.g.* a cut with soil contamination may possibly be infected with tetanus

bacilli). There is no time to wait while his body makes
the necessary antibodies and antitoxins, therefore he is
given large doses of serum which already contains them.
The serum is taken from an animal, usually a horse,
that has been immunized by vaccine injections. Since
the patient's body has taken no part in the process this
is called **passive immunity**. The effect of the injections
is not lasting, but the body is given time in which to
develop its own reactions. In some cases the serum for
injection is taken from someone who has just recovered
from the disease.

Susceptibility Tests

These tests are useful in the event of an outbreak of
diphtheria or scarlet fever in a school, to discover which
of the children who are contacts are liable to develop
the disease. In some schools a susceptibility test for
tuberculosis is done on all children when they first
enter, and in many hospitals the test is done on student
nurses when they enter the Preliminary Training School.

Diphtheria—The Schick Test.

The purpose is to show if an individual is immune to
diphtheria. A minute dose of diphtheria toxin is injected into the skin of the forearm (intradermal injection). If he is immune there will be no reaction since
there are antibodies in the blood to destroy the toxin.
If susceptible there will be a positive reaction—a red
inflamed area round the site of injection. These individuals may then be immunized.

Scarlet Fever—The Dick Test.

Susceptibility to scarlet fever is discovered by an
intradermal injection of toxin of the hæmolytic streptococcus that causes the disease. A red inflamed area, or
positive reaction, shows that the individual has no antibodies to destroy that toxin and is therefore not immune.

Tuberculosis—see p. 283.

Forms of Vaccination and Immunization

Vaccination against smallpox is advised when the infant is 3 or 4 months old. It is not compulsory, but if the parents ignore the advisory letter sent by the Medical Officer of Health, the health visitor sees them and tries to persuade them to bring the baby to the clinic or take him to their own doctor.

Calf lymph vaccine is used, and a repeat is given during school years.

Immunization against diphtheria is advised when the child is about 10 months old. An injection of toxoid is given (A.P.T.—alum precipitated toxoid) followed in four weeks' time by another bigger dose. Antibodies are formed which confer immunity. Before he goes to school and later when at school, he is given a boosting dose; this time of T.A.F. (toxoid antitoxin floccules). This is *active immunization*.

Since immunization was introduced the incidence of diphtheria has decreased rapidly. Parents are persuaded to bring their children to be immunized by means of talks given by health visitors, display posters, and other forms of publicity.

Passive immunity is needed only when the patient is actually suffering from diphtheria. Large doses of diphtheria anti-toxin are then injected to provide him with antibodies to overcome the infection.

Whooping Cough [Pertussis]. To immunize a baby he may be given three injections at intervals of one month. This is done when he is about six months old.

Poliomyelitis. Vaccination of children is at the parents' choice.

Typhoid and Paratyphoid Fever. Vaccination is necessary for all who are going to countries where sanitation is bad, and where water and food are liable to be contaminated.

Tetanus. Soldiers and others who are liable to suffer dirt contamination in wounds are inoculated against tetanus by injections of formol-toxoid. This produces an *active* immunity. All patients with wounds and abrasions that may be infected from the soil are given injections of tetanus antitoxin. This is *passive* immunity.

VENEREAL DISEASES

These diseases include syphilis and gonorrhœa. Over the years they have cost the nation much in many ways; the birth rate is lowered due to sterility and abortions; much ill-health is caused and working efficiency is therefore lowered; children may be infected, as with congenital syphilis, or they may become blind due to ophthalmia neonatorum—*i.e.* (gonorrheal) infection of the eyes of the newborn.

Compulsory notification has not been adopted in this country, except in the case of ophthalmia neonatorum, which is "purulent discharge from the eyes commencing within twenty-one days from the date of birth".

The midwife is required to call in medical aid for "any inflammation of, or discharge from, the eyes, however slight", and to notify the Local Supervising Authority.

This notification, together with certain precautions taken at the birth of the baby, is for the purpose of safeguarding the baby's sight, since every case at once receives intensive treatment.

In clinics for venereal disease, which are free and confidential, modern treatments result in a high percentage of cures.

TUBERCULOSIS

This has caused in past years a very heavy death rate. It is notifiable in all forms. There are two types of tubercle bacillus, the human and the bovine, and the sources and results of infection are:

| Tuberculosis of lung. | Human type usually. | From sputum, articles contaminated with sputum, kissing, dust (since the bacillus can live dried). |
| Surgical tuberculosis—*i.e.*, bones, joints, glands, etc. | Bovine type usually. | Milk from tuberculous cows given to babies. |

The disease is not hereditary but very young children easily acquire it from milk or from their parents. Overcrowded dwellings, poor food, and lack of sunlight are predisposing factors.

Workers in "dusty trades", especially those dealing with stone containing much silica, are predisposed to tuberculosis of the lungs due to irritation by inhaled particles.

Measures to Control Pulmonary Tuberculosis

Tuberculosis was made notifiable in 1912 since when the Medical Officer of Health has been responsible for tracing the source of infection in each case and assessing the suitability of the patient's environment. Tuberculosis Officers were appointed later and dispensaries established, and in 1943 mass radiography was introduced. In 1949 B.C.G. vaccination of contacts was first used in the United Kingdom. The intensive campaign against tuberculosis has brought encouraging results. The number of cases notified has fallen consistently in the last ten years and the number of deaths shows a spectacular drop. This improvement has been

10*

brought about by the vigorous and concentrated work
of the **Tuberculosis Team** consisting of:

The Chest Physician (Tuberculosis Officer).
Tuberculosis Health Visitor.
Tuberculosis Almoner.
Mass Radiography Units.
Disablement Resettlement Officers.
Care Committees.
The Sanitary Inspector in connection with
housing inspection.

When an early case has been diagnosed, the patient
attends at a tuberculosis dispensary. Here he comes
under the care of the Tuberculosis Officer who will
decide whether he shall remain in his home, or be put
on the waiting list for a bed in a sanatorium or be sent
to a chest hospital. All contacts in the patient's home,
place of work, etc., are asked to attend for mass radiography so that early cases may be discovered and treated.

If the patient is to remain at home he is under the
care of his own doctor and attends at the dispensary at
intervals.

The Tuberculosis Visitor (see p. 236) will visit him
frequently and will see that he understands the use of
his sputum flask, the danger of spreading infection and
how it may be avoided.

Patients who return to their homes from sanatoria
are kept under observation in the same way.

It is for these cases that Care Committees do so much.
They are voluntary organizations, and consequently
free from official restrictions, and are frequently able to
supplement by various means all that the health and
welfare services have achieved for the patient. Often it
is to their interest and help that the ex-patient owes his
opportunity to make a fresh start with new interest in
life. For cases in which return home is not advised
there are colonies where the patients may work at a

trade and live with their families in houses in the settlement, remaining always under supervision of a doctor.

Susceptibility Tests

(*a*) **The Tuberculin Jelly Test** is useful for children. Tuberculin jelly is applied on a small area between the shoulder blades and covered with adhesive strapping. On a similar area control jelly is applied and covered. The strapping is removed in forty-eight hours.

A positive reaction is shown by a red area with papules where the diagnostic jelly was applied. This may mean either that the child has active tuberculosis or, probably, that he has developed immunity through having been in contact with someone who has the disease in an infectious form.

The child would be examined at the chest clinic and contacts sought out and asked to attend the mass radiography clinic. Those with a negative reaction may be vaccinated with B.C.G.

(*b*) **The Mantoux Test.** A minute dose of the toxin of tubercle bacilli is injected intradermally in the front of the forearm.

A negative reaction shows that the person has not at any time been infected with tubercle bacilli. If he is then vaccinated with B.C.G. he will develop an active immunity.

A positive reaction—a raised red area—shows that he has, or in the past has had, infection with tubercle bacilli. He would be referred to the chest clinic for investigation and treatment if necessary. Contacts would be asked to attend also for investigation.

B.C.G. [Bacillus Calmette-Guérin] Vaccination

In November 1953, the Ministry of Health, in a circular issued to Local Authorities, approved vaccination of school children against tuberculosis during their last year at school when over 13 years of age. Permission to vaccinate children of a lower age group is awaiting the results of trials now being undertaken by the Medical Research Council. Where the policy is adopted the responsibility for arranging the procedure will rest with the Medical Officer of Health and the School Medical Officer. The purpose of B.C.G. vaccination is explained to the parents and their consent is obtained in writing. If the child or adult has a negative Mantoux or tuberculin jelly test this shows that he has not been infected with tubercle bacilli and therefore his tissues have not been stimulated to produce antibodies and he needs to be vaccinated.

The medical examination of medical students and nurses, all of whom are liable to come in contact with tuberculous patients, includes chest X-ray and a Mantoux test. Those who are non-reactors have the test repeated with a stronger solution, and if there is still no reaction they are vaccinated with B.C.G.

The Control of Surgical Tuberculosis

The provision of a "safe" milk for children is the chief means by which the disease has been reduced in so spectacular manner. "Tuberculin Tested (Pasteurized)" is the best milk obtainable for children. Welfare centres provide safe milk at a reduced cost.

THE CONTROL OF GASTRO-ENTERITIS IN BABIES

In the last half century the death rate of infants from gastro-enteritis during the first year of life has fallen to one-fourth of the previous figure.

This is largely due to the effective measures taken to prevent the spread of infection together with more efficient social services, and to the use for artificial feeds of dried milks which are not liable to be contaminated by flies.

The infection is passed from excreta of the infants and from their napkins and cot linen, to the hands of those in charge of them, and so to bottles, teats and feeds. Flies may pass on the infection in the same way.

Strict technique has checked the spread. In infants' hospitals the baby is isolated, and all toilet and feed articles are kept separate and washed separately. Feeds are prepared by a nurse who does not handle the baby and should on no account be given by one who changes him. Bottles, teats and measures are washed by the feed nurse with special care in the routine method, boiled and kept covered in the boiled water or in Milton solution, the teats being kept dry in a sterile container. The technique of gowns, masks and hand-washing is, of course, strictly carried out.

Instruction given by health visitors and midwives to mothers, both at infant welfare clinics and in the homes, is an important factor in the virtual disappearance of "summer diarrhoea".

INTERNATIONAL CONTROL OF INFECTIOUS DISEASES

Information with regard to outbreaks of infectious diseases is supplied to all countries from the Head-quarters of World Health Organization now at Copenhagen.

CONTROL OF INFECTIOUS DISEASES AT AIRPORTS

Special precautions are taken with regard to smallpox, plague, cholera, yellow fever and typhus fever.

The Commander of an incoming aircraft hands to the Medical Officer a signed Declaration of Health, and in the event of there being a suspected case on board, the Medical Officer may examine the patient and, if he thinks necessary, detain the aircraft.

If an aircraft has come from, or called at an airport in a place where infection has been notified, every passenger receives a yellow card with instructions to report to his doctor at once if he feels ill within 21 days. He hands the yellow card to the doctor who must if he suspects such illness, notify the Medical Officer of Health at once by telephone.

Should a person having travelled by air develop one of the above diseases within 21 days the fact is broadcast so that the other passengers who travelled on the aeroplane may be warned.

CONTROL OF INFECTIOUS DISEASES AT SEA PORTS

A Port Medical Officer of Health receives from the Ministry of Health a list of ports from which cases of infectious disease have been reported. He must inspect all vessels on arriving from such ports.

He must also inspect any vessel having on board an infected or suspected person, the master of the ship having notified him before arrival.

The Medical Officer has further powers concerning the examination of persons intending to embark whom he suspects of being infected with the scheduled diseases. (See above.)

The master of every ship must hand a signed Declaration of Health to the port officials on arrival.

VITAL STATISTICS

Notification of Births Act. The birth of a child (alive or dead) must be notified to the M.O.H. within thirty-six hours, both by the father (if residing in the house) and the person attending at the birth.

(Registration of birth is additional to the above, and is made within six weeks to the Registrar of Births, Marriages and Deaths.)

Vital statistics show by means of figures and graphs the variations in birth rate, death rate, infant mortality, maternal mortality, occupational mortality, incidence of various diseases, etc. They are compiled from reports and returns made to the Ministry of Health.

During the present century statistics have shown some remarkable results.

Both maternal and infant mortality decreased greatly in the ten years from 1938. The figures per 1000 births are:

	Maternal Mortality	Infant Mortality
1938	3·25	53
1948	1·02	34

The big drop in maternal mortality is due to ante-natal care and to chemotherapy in cases of puerperal sepsis. The drop in infant mortality continues the progress made during the last fifty years since the introduction of the maternal and child welfare services and is undoubtedly due to these and to improving standards of living. Diphtheria, measles and scarlet fever all show a spectacular decline. The figure for lung tuberculosis during the last fifty years is reduced to about one-half, and "surgical" tuberculosis to one-fifth.

TRANSMISSION OF INFECTIOUS DISEASES

The following table shows the modes of transmission of the common infectious diseases. Methods to prevent transmission, and also incubation and isolation periods, are included for reference.

Disease.	Incuba-tion.	Prevention of Spread.	Infectious Material—Special Precautions.	Isolation.	Quarantine for Contacts.
Scarlet fever.	2–5 days.	Notification. Isolation. Exclusion of contacts from school. Immunization of contacts if Dick positive. Investigation of milk supply.	Discharges from ear, nose, throat, handkerchiefs, swabs, etc., burnt or disinfected.	4 weeks or till no discharge.	10 days.
Measles.	10–14 days.	Isolation if possible. Exclusion of contacts from school. Passive immunization of contacts with serum from convalescents.	As above.	2 weeks.	16 days.
German measles.	14–18 days.	Isolation if possible.	Nose and throat secretions: care as above.	1 week.	3 weeks.
Diphtheria.	2–4 days.	Notification. Isolation. Exclusion of contacts from school. Supervision of contacts: swabs taken and cultured, immunized with serum if Schick positive. Search for and isolation of carriers. Investigation of milk supply.	Nose and throat secretions: care as above.	Till three negative swabs at 2-day intervals.	If Schick positive, prophylactic vaccination.

Whooping-cough.	8–10 days.	Isolation if possible.	Nose and throat secretions, sputum and vomit.	6 weeks.	3 weeks.
Mumps.	17–21 days.	Isolation.	Nose and throat secretions.	3 weeks.	3 weeks.
Enteric fever (typhoid and paratyphoid fevers).	7–21 days.	Notification. Strict barrier nursing. Investigation of water supply. Investigation of milk supply. Investigation of drainage. Search for carriers. Boiling of suspected water or closure of wells. Killing flies and covering food. Prophylactic immunization (with a vaccine of typhoid and paratyphoid A and B organisms).	Stools and urine. Fomites — especially bedpan, urinals, bed linen. Disinfection of all these and lavatory or sluice.	Till there have been three consecutive negative cultures for *Salmonella typhosa* and *S. paratyphi* in faeces and urine.	
Typhus fever.	12 days.	Notification. Barrier nursing. Thorough disinfection of patient's home, bedding and clothes. Destruction of lice, fleas and bugs. Supervision of contacts, with disinfestation of any who are verminous. A disease of dirty conditions.	Destruction of lice, etc. Patient's clothing fumigated or burnt.	4 weeks.	2 weeks.

Disease.	Incubation.	Prevention of Spread.	Infectious Material—Special Precautions.	Isolation.	Quarantine for Contacts.
Smallpox.	12–14 days.	Notification. Isolation in special hospitals. Vaccination and revaccination when cases occur. Following up contacts for revaccination and quarantine. Supervision of ships' crews, tramps, etc. Notification of schools and workshops. Following up suspicious cases. Disinfection of patients' clothes, house, and places he visited. Chickenpox made notifiable. Nurses in charge of patients isolated also.	Skin and epithelial scales, scabs and crusts. Secretions of mouth and nose and all fomites.	Till every scab is gone.	21 days.
Chickenpox.	17 days.	Isolation. Notification only when smallpox is about.	Droplets from nose and throat. Fluid from broken vesicles, even when dried.	Till all scabs are gone.	3 weeks.
Cerebrospinal meningitis.	1–5 days.	Notification. Isolation. Search for carriers (swabs from nasopharynx cultured). Antiseptic gargles for contacts and carriers.	Nose and throat secretions.	Till 1 week after temperature is normal.	10 days.

		Notification.	Probably droplets from nose and throat.		7 days.
Encephalitis lethargica.	1–7 days.				
Erysipelas.	1–4 days.	Notification. Barrier nursing.	Wound discharges and dressings.		14 days.
Poliomyelitis (infantile paralysis).	5–10 days.	Notification. Barrier nursing. Disinfection of stools. Postponement to inter-epidemic periods of operations on ear, nose and throat for all possible contacts.	Nose and throat secretions infectious, though dried. Stools.	21 days.	14 days.
Dysentery: (a) Bacillary; (b) Amoebic.	2–8 days. —	Notification. Barrier nursing. Investigation of water and milk supplies. Search for carriers, especially in (a). Vaccination in (b). Killing flies and covering food.	Stools and urine. Fomites, especially bedpan, urinals and bed linen. Disinfection of all these and lavatory or sluice.	Till 1 week after temperature and stools are normal and two consecutive stool cultures are negative.	
Epidemic diarrhoea (summer diarrhoea).	1–2 days.	Covering food, especially babies' feeds, from flies. Killing flies. Use of dried milk in place of condensed for babies. Cleanliness of sanitary arrangements. Clearing up of all dirt and refuse.	Stools, and fomites contaminated therewith.		

Disease.	Incubation.	Prevention of Spread.	Infectious Material— Special Precautions.	Isolation.	Quarantine for Contacts.
Malaria.	8–10 days.	Notification. Draining of all stagnant water if possible. Spraying ponds with kerosene. Destruction of mosquitoes. Use of mosquito nets.			
Influenza.	1–4 days.	Avoidance of crowded places. Sufficient "protective foods" in diet. (See Chap. IX.) Gargles.	Nose and throat secretions.	Till temperature is normal and patient is free from discharges.	7 days.
Tuberculosis, all types.		Notification. Laws against expectoration in public places. Better housing and less overcrowding. Sanatorium treatment. Tuberculosis dispensaries for advice and treatment. Village colonies. Open-air schools. Health visiting for home advice. Meat inspection. Milk grading. B.C.G. vaccination of child contacts if Tuberculin tests are negative.	Sputum (pulmonary type): Use of flask. Use of paper handkerchiefs and burn. Patient taught: To cover the mouth with handkerchief when coughing, to wash hands after using handkerchief when possible, not to kiss people, especially children.		

Disease	Period	Preventive Measures	Infective Material		
Syphilis.	2–6 weeks.	Treatment in free confidential clinics. Care in use of public lavatories.	All discharges.		
Gonorrhœa.	3–6 days.	Avoidance of public towels, cups, etc. Education of the public.	All discharges.		
Ophthalmia neonatorum. (Infection of eyes of new-born baby with gonococcus.)	3 days.	Notification. Isolation of baby and all utensils. Prophylaxis: antenatal treatment of mother if infected. treatment of baby's eyes at birth. care with towels, sponges, bed linen, etc.	Discharge from eyes.		

INDEX

INDEX

Abortus fever, 193
Acarus scabiei, 147
Acne, 97
Activated sludge, 88
Aeration tank, 88
Aged, care of, 234, 271–3
Air, circulation, 12, 13
  composition, 9, 10
  conditioned, 29
  contamination in wards, 18
  humidity, 12
  pollution, 13–18
  pressure, 10
  temperature, 11, 12
  space required, 20
Airports, control of infection, 285
Almoner, 239
Antenatal clinic, 224–8
Anthrax, 125
Antibodies, 276–7
Anti-siphonage pipe, 80–1
Arnott's ventilator, 27
Artesian wells, 64
Artificial feeding, 107–8
  lighting, 53–8
Ascorbic acid, 180
Atmosphere, 9
  composition, 9, 10
  currents, 12, 13
  humidity, 12
  temperature, 11, 12
  pollution, 13–18
Atmospheric pressure, 10, 11

Baby, feeding of, 107–8
  hygiene of, 108–10
Background heating, 37, 39, 47–51
Bacteria, 124–7
  classification of, 124, 126
  destruction of, 131–2
  in air, 14, 18, 129
  in food, 202–4
  in milk, 192–3
Balance system of ventilation, 25

Balanced diet, 184–5
Barometer, 11
Barrier nursing, 136
Baths, 79, 97
  babies', 108
B.C.G. vaccination, 283–4
Beetles, 167–8
Benefits (National Insurance), 243
Beri-beri, 179
Beveridge report, 241–2
Bins, refuse, 93, 212
Biological filters, 87–8
Blackheads, 97
Blind, training of, 256–7
Body, temperature, regulation of, 119
Botulism, 203
Bowels, action of, 103
  in babies, 109
  in pregnancy, 226
  in toddlers, 112
Breathing, 102
Bromidrosis, 99
Bugs, 153
Bunions, 99

Calcium in food, 173
  in water, 74
Calorie values, 182–4
Camping, 114–16
Candles, 58
Canning of food, 204–5
Carbohydrates, 171–2
Carbon dioxide, 9, 10, 14, 207
  monoxide, 14, 15, 268
Carotene, 176
Carriers, 128, 129, 275, 289, 291
Catchment area, 61
Central heating, 47–51, 39
Cesspools, 90
Chemical treatment of sewage, 93
Chickenpox, 290
Child guidance clinic, 248, 249
  minders, 245

Children Act, 244, 245
  adopted, 244
  foster, 244
  one to five years, 110–13
  school age, 251–61
Children's Charter, 244
  Officer, 244
Chlorination of water, 68
Cisterns, 73
Citizens' Advice Bureau, 240–1
Cleanliness, personal, 96–102
Clothing, 119–23
  of baby, 108, 109
  and body temperature, 119–120
  of toddler, 111–12
  for camping, 114–16
Coal, combustion products, 14–18
  gas, 42–3
  tar derivatives, 43
Cockroaches, 167, 213
Cold storage, 205–7
Colour, 51
Combustion products, 14–18
Comedones, 97
Communicable diseases, 128
  spread of, 129, 130, 275, 288–93
  control of, 274–86
Conditioned air, 29
Conduction of heat, 36, 37
Conservancy system of sewage disposal, 92
Constipation, 103
Contacts, 128, 275
Contamination of air, 13–19
  of food, 201–4
  of milk, 192, 193
  of water, 59, 91
Convection of heat, 35, 36
  currents, winds, 12, 13, 22
Cooper's disc, 24, 25
Copper in food, 174
Corns, 99
Cotton, 122
County Borough Councils, 215, 218
  Councils, 215, 218
Cross ventilation, 23

Damp-proof course, 3, 4
Deaf, training of, 257

Deep-freezing, 207
Dehydrated food, 205
  milk, 200
Delicate children, schools for, 258
Deprived children, 234
Detritus tank, 86
Diarrhœa, infantile, 129, 130, 284, 285, 291
Diesel oil, combustion products, 15
Diet, antenatal, 225
  balanced, 184
  deficiency diseases, 177–82
  in old age, 118
  of toddler, 111
  requirements, 169, 182
Diphtheria, immunization against, 279
  and milk, 193
  prevention of spread, 288
  Schick test, 278
Diseases, deficiency, 177–82
  infectious, control of, 274–286
  spread of, 129, 130, 288–293
  occupational, 267–9
  spread by carriers, 129
  by food, 130, 202
  by milk, 129, 193
  by water, 59, 91, 129
Disinfection, current, 134
  methods of, 131–4
  terminal, 135
  of verminous premises, 134, 135
Distillation, 66, 67
District Nurse, 237–9
Domestic filter, 67
Drain-house, 83
Drainage laws, 222
  chemical system, 93
  conservancy system, 92, 93
  water-carriage system, 76–85
Droplet infection, 18, 129
Dust, 18, 19
  and occupational diseases, 268
  borne diseases, 130
Dysentery, Amœba of, 162
  prevention of spread, 204–214, 291

Dysentery, spread of, 59, 91, 129, 130, 202

Earth closets, 92
Effluent of sewage, 87
purification of, 87, 88
Electricity, 44–6
Electric heaters, 46
lighting, 54–7
Electro-magnetic waves, 31–4
Enteric fever—see typhoid fever
Environment, 261–2
Excreta, disposal of, 76–93
Exercise, 104
during pregnancy, 227
of baby, 110
of toddler, 112
Extraction and exhaust fans, 24, 266, 268, 269

Fabrics, 120–3
Factories, welfare in, 264–7
Fatigue, 104, 105
Fats, 172
Feet, care of, 98–100
Feeding of baby, 107
artificial, 107, 108
mixed, 108
Fermentation, 125, 146, 202
Filter beds, 69
Filters, domestic, 67
pressure, 69, 70
Filtration of water, 67, 69–70
of effluent, 87
of air, 29
Fires, coal and wood, 41, 42
gas, 42, 44
Flats, 7
Fleas, human, 150
rat, 151–3
Flies, 162–4, 213
Fluorine, 174
Fog, 17, 18
Food, contamination of, 201–204, 209, 210
diseases spread by, 202
and Drugs Act, 210
in the home, 206, 207, 208, 213, 214
hygiene, 210–14

Food poisoning, 203, 204, 209, 210
preservation, 204–8
requirements, 169, 182–5
substances and uses, 169–82
Foster children, 234, 244
Fumes, 18

Garchey system of refuse disposal, 94
Gases, in atmosphere, 13
of combustion, 14
Gas fires, 42
Gastro-enteritis in babies, 284, 285, 291

Habits, 106, 110, 112
Hands, care of, 98
Hardness of water, 74, 75
Head, care of, 100
Health Visitor, 229–37
Heat, nature of, 34–7
preservation of food by, 204, 205
transmission of, 35–7
treatment of milk, 197–200
Heaters, oil, 44
electric, 46
gas, 42, 44
Heating the house, methods, 37–51
background, 37, 39, 44, 46, 47–51
Hinckes-Bird ventilation method, 24, 25
Home Help, 239
Home Nursing Service, 237–9
Home Office, 220
and Approved Schools, 246–8
Hookworm, 156
Hopper sash, 24, 27
House drain, 83
planning, 3–8
Household refuse, 93–5
Housing Acts, 222
Humidity, atmospheric, 12
Humidifying of air, 29
Humus tank, 88
Hydrocyanic acid gas, 134
Hygiene of ward, 137–9
of sick room, 139–41
Hygrometer, 12

Immunity, 276–8
Immunization, 279
Incineration, 94, 95
Incubation and quarantine, 127, 288–93
Industrial diseases, 267–9
Infant mortality, 287
welfare clinic, 232, 233
Infection, 124–30
Infectious diseases, 288–93
notification of, 128
at airports, 285, 286
at seaports, 286
prevention and control of, 274–93
spread of, 129, 288–93
Inspection chamber, 83
Insulation of buildings, 3
of refrigerators, 207
heat, 4, 37–9
sound, 4, 7
Intercepting chamber and trap, 83–5
Iodine, 174
Iron in food, 174
Isotopes, 31

Kata˙thermometer, 28

Lactic acid bacillus, 192
Lagging of pipes, 40, 41
Land treatment of sewage, 90
Lead in water, 60
Lice, 148–50
Light, 51–2
Lighting, artificial, 53–8
natural, 52–3
Linen, 122
disinfection of, 133
Local authorities, 215, 217, 219
Health Authorities, 215, 216, 218
Louvred panes, 24, 26, 53

Magnesium, 174
Malaria, 164, 292
Margarine, 172
Materials, 120–3
Maternal mortality, 287
Maternity Nurse, 228
Services, 224–9

McKinnel's roof ventilator, 26
Measles, prevention of spread, 288
"Measly" pork, 157
Meat, 170
contamination of, 203, 209
inspection, 211
preservation, 204, 205, 207
Medical Officer of Health, 220, 221
of Ports, 286
Mental defectives, 249, 250
Metabolism and diet, 181–5
Midwife, the, 228
Milk, 185–200
bacteria in, 192, 193
clean, regulations for, 188–192
composition of, 186, 187
diseases spread by, 193, 129
dried, 200
from attested herds, 194, 195
grading and designations, 194
pasteurization, 197–9
safe, regulations for, 192, 193
tuberculin tested, 195–7
Mineral salts in food, 173
in water, 59, 74
Ministry of Health, 217, 218, 219
Ministries concerned with health, 216–20
Mosquitoes, 164–6
Motor spirit, exhaust gases of, 14, 15
Moths, 167
Moulds, 142, 143, 201
Mouth, care of, 100
Mumps, spread of, 289

Nails, 98
National Assistance Act, 241
Health Service Act, 217, 218, 241
Insurance Act, 241
Natural purification of water, 68
ventilation, 21–4
helps to, 24–7
Nicotinic acid, 179

Nitrifying bacteria, 125, 126
Nitrogen, 10
Notifiable diseases, 128
Notification of births, 286
Nuisances, 223
Nylon, 122

Occupational diseases and accidents, 267–70
    health, 264–71
    nurse, 265, 266
    rehabilitation 270, 271
Offensive trades, 223
Oil lamps, 58
    heaters 44
Old age, care in, 116
Orientation of houses, 2
Oxygen, 9, 13
Ozone, in purification of water, 70

Panel and Panelite heating, 50
Parasites, 142–62
Paronychia, 98
Pasteur - Chamberland filter, 67
Pasteurization, 197–9
Pediculi, 148–50
Pellagra, 179
Percolating filters, 87, 88
Perflation, 22
Permutit process for water softening, 75
Personal hygiene, 96–106
Personnel of Health Services, 220–41
Phosphorus, 174
Physical fitness, 102–6
Pipes, anti-siphonage, 80, 81
    soil, 79, 82
    water, 80, 82
Plague, 151
Play, 112
Plenum system of ventilation, 24
Poliomyelitis, 129, 291
Pollution of atmosphere, 13–18
    of water, 59, 60, 91, 92
Ports, control of infection, 151, 286

Potassium, 174
Preservation of food, 204–8
Pressure, atmospheric, 10, 11
    filters, 69
Prevention of infectious diseases, 274–86
Privies, 92
Products of combustion, 14–18
Protein foods, 170, 171
Protozoa, 126
Public Health Acts, 215, 216
    Inspector, 221–2
Pulex irritans, 150
Purification of swimming baths, 70
    of water, 66–70
Putrefaction, 125
Pyridoxin, 180

Queen's Nurses, 237–9

Radiation, 31–4, 35
Radio-active decay, 31
Rain water, 66
Rat fleas, 151
Rats, 151–3, 168
Recreation, 105, 114–16, 256, 260, 263, 264
Refrigeration, 206, 207
Refuse, 93, 94
    disposal, 94, 95
    Garchey system, 94
Regional Hospital Boards, 217
Reservoirs, storage, 68
    service, 72
Respiration, products of, 13, 14
Rest, 104, 105
Rheumatism, 262, 263
Riboflavine, 179
Rickets, 178
Ringworm, 143, 146
Roberts's separator, 66
Roofs, 5, 38
Roof insulation, 38
Roughage, 103, 174
Roundworms, 154

Salmonella, 203, 209, 210, 211, 212

Salting of food, 205
Salts in food, 172–4
Sand filtration of water, 69–70
Sanitary laws, 222–3
Sanitation, 76–93
Saprophytes, 125
Scabies, 147–8
Scarlet fever, prevention of spread, 288
  Dick Test, 278
School, approved, 245–8
  child, 113–16
  county primary, 251, 252
    secondary, 251–4
  health service, 258–60
  meals, 259–60
  Medical Officer, 258, 261
  Nurse, 260, 261
  nursery, 254, 256
  special, 256–8
Schick Test, 278
Scurvy, 181
Seborrhœa, 100
Sedimentation tanks, 86, 87
Sewage, 76–93
  activated sludge method, 88
  disposal of, 85–93
  cesspool system, 91
  chemical treatment, 90, 93
  conservancy system, 92, 93
  contamination of water, 91, 92
  land treatment, 90
  percolating filter, 87, 88
  preliminary treatment, 86, 87
Sewer, 85
Sherringham valve, 24, 26
Shoes, 100
Short circuit, 45
Silk, 122
Skin, cleanliness of, 96–8
  and sunlight, 106
Slaughterhouses, 211
Sleep, 104, 105, 109, 112
Sludge, activated, 88
  disposal of, 88, 90
Smallpox, prevention of spread, 290
  vaccination against, 279
Smoke, 15–18
Smoking of food, 205
Soap, action of, 97

Social Medicine and Insurance, 241
Sodium, 173
Softening of water, 74
Soil pipe, 82
Space heating, large scale, 47–51
  small scale, 39
Spore-forming bacilli, 125
  moulds, 143
Springs, 65
Sputum containers, 134
  diseases spread by, 130, 289, 292
Staphylococci in food, 204
Steam disinfection, 131
Sulphur dioxide, 14, 15
  salts in food, 174
  in water, 74
Sunlight, effects of, 106
Susceptibility tests, 278, 283
Swimming baths, 70, 71

Tanks, aeration, 88
  humus, 88, 89
  sedimentation, 87, 89
  septic, 91
  water, 72, 73
Tapeworms, 158–62
  beef, 158, 159
  dog, 161, 162
  pork, 151, 161
Teeth, 101, 102, 110, 226
  fluorine in, 174
Temperature of atmosphere, 11
Terminal disinfection, 135, 136
Threadworms, 155, 156
Thrush, 146
Ticks, 154
Tinea, 143
Tips, refuse, 94, 95
Tobins tubes, 24, 27
Toddlers, 110–13
Town Planning, 1–3
Traps in drainage system, 77–83
Tuberculosis, 280–4
  control of, 281–4, 292
  and milk, 195–7
  vaccination against, 283, 284
  visitor, 236, 237

Typhoid fever and ice cream, 210
  and milk, 193
  prevention of spread, 289
  spread of, 129, 130
  and water, 59, 91, 92
Typhus fever, 149, 289

Ultra-violet rays, 33, 177
Upland surface water, 60–2

Vaccination, 279
Venereal diseases, 280, 293
Ventilation, 19–29
  in factories, 266
  helps to, 24–7
  mechanical, 24–9
  natural, 21–4
  test for efficiency, 27–9
Vermin, destruction of, 168, 212
Vital statistics, 286–7
Vitamins, 175–82

Walls, structure of, 3–5
Ward, hygiene of, 137–41
Water, 59–75
  balance in body, 175
  chlorination of, 68

Water, distribution of, 72–4
  drinking, 59
  filtration, 67, 69, 70
  ground and damp-proof course, 3
  laws relating to, 223
  pipes, 72, 82
  pollution of, 59, 60, 129
  purification of, 66–71
  softening of, 74
  sources of, 60–6
  supply of a country, 60
  vapour, 10, 14
Water-carriage system of drainage, 76–85
Waterproof material, 123
Waves, electro-magnetic, 31–4
Wells, 62–5
Whooping cough, immunization against, 279
  prevention of spread, 289
Windows, types of, 52, 53
Wiring, electric, 45, 46
Wool, 121, 122
World Health Organization, 285
Worms, 154–62

Yeasts, 146, 202

Zeolite, 75

Printed in Great Britain
SPOTTISWOODE, BALLANTYNE & CO. LTD.
London and Colchester

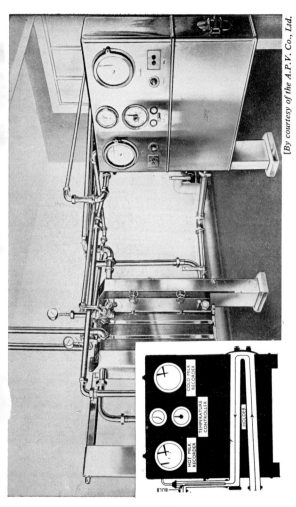

[By courtesy of the A.P.V. Co., Ltd.

FIG. 71.—A modern pasteurization plant—H.T.S.T. (High Temperature Short Time) method. (For description see page 197.) Inset shows in section the Holding Tube in the Control Panel, where the milk is heated as it flows.

305

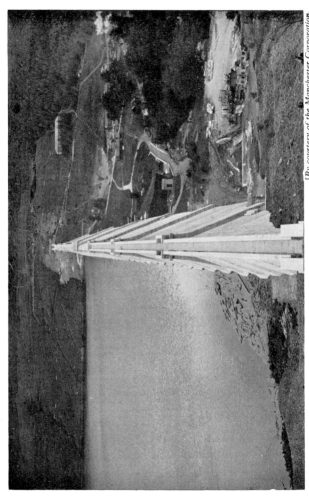

FIG. 73. Haweswater Dam, Westmorland, one of the three sources of Manchester's water supply.

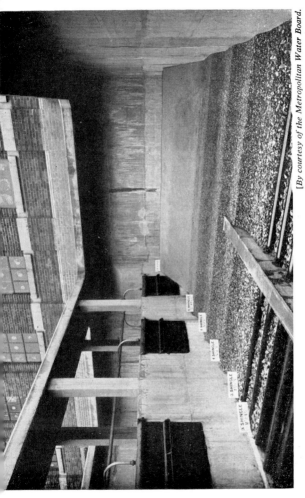

[By courtesy of the Metropolitan Water Board.]

Fig. 73.—Section through a rapid primary filter.

These filters remove coarse particles, so relieving the slow secondary filters. They are cleaned daily so no zooglea layer forms, but there are, within the sand, bacteria that oxidize any traces of ammonia present.

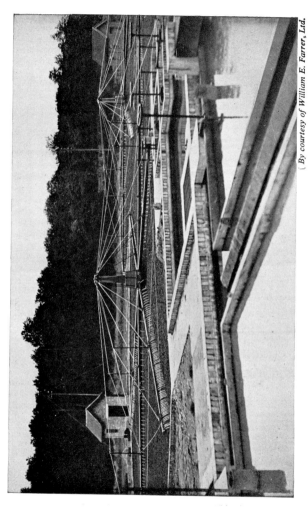

By courtesy of William E. Farrer, Ltd.

FIG. 74.— Sewage disposal works, showing sedimentation tanks and percolating filters.

308

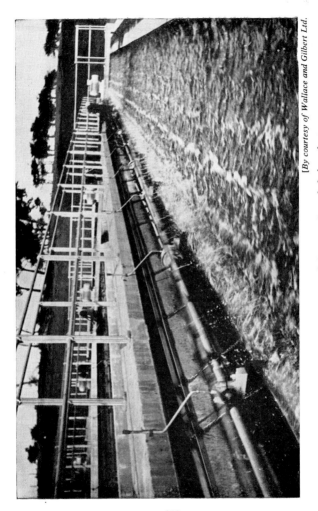

Fig. 75.—*Aeration tank in an activated sludge plant.*

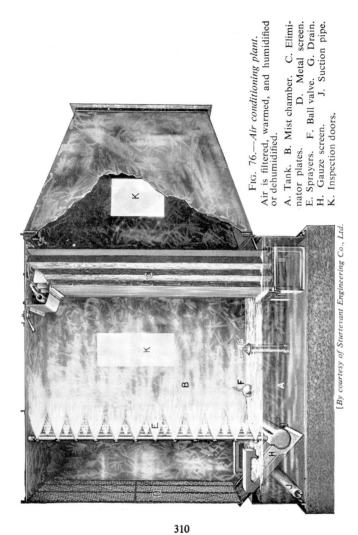

FIG. 76.—*Air conditioning plant.*
Air is filtered, warmed, and humidified or dehumidified.

A. Tank. B. Mist chamber. C. Eliminator plates. D. Metal screen. E. Sprayers. F. Ball valve. G. Drain. H. Gauze screen. J. Suction pipe. K. Inspection doors.

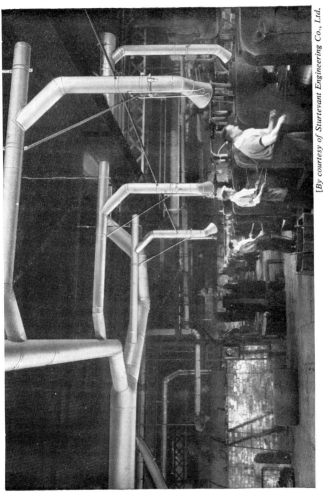

[By courtesy of *Sturtevant Engineering Co., Ltd.*]

FIG. 77.—*Cold air douche plant to apply cooling air to men in the rolling mills.*

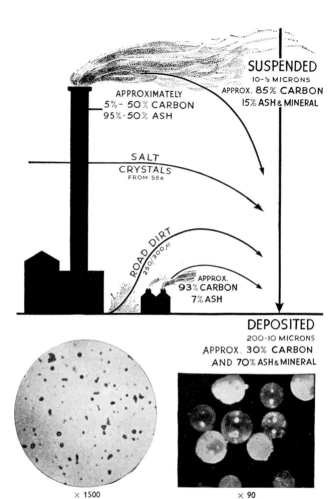

SUSPENDED
10-½ MICRONS
APPROX. 85% CARBON
15% ASH & MINERAL

APPROXIMATELY
5% - 50% CARBON
95% - 50% ASH

SALT
CRYSTALS
FROM SEA

ROAD DIRT
250/300 μ

APPROX.
93% CARBON
7% ASH

DEPOSITED
200-10 MICRONS
APPROX. 30% CARBON
AND 70% ASH & MINERAL

× 1500

× 90

FIG. 78.—*Atmospheric pollution.*
The upper illustration shows diagrammatically some of the features of
atmospheric pollution. The lower illustrations show (left) the very
minute particles found suspended in the atmosphere and (right) boiler
flue grit which is much coarser and will be deposited.

Nurses' Aids Series

This Series is designed to provide complete textbooks covering the various fields of knowledge required by the student nurse. It covers the subjects included in the syllabus of the General Nursing Council and, in addition, volumes on certain specialised subjects such as ophthalmic nursing, ear, nose and throat nursing, the setting of trays and trolleys, and theatre technique are included. New volumes are added to the Series from time to time, and each book is kept fully up to date in new editions.

Each volume is a complete textbook on its subject and is written by a Sister Tutor at a well-known hospital. The whole Series aims at providing concisely, clearly and simply just that amount of information which the nurse needs to possess, gathered together in easily read and easily carried, well illustrated volumes at a price within the means of any nurse.

A list of the volumes available in the Series will be found on the next page. New volumes or new editions may have been added since this list was printed; up-to-date information will gladly be supplied by

THE SALES DEPARTMENT

BAILLIÈRE, TINDALL AND COX

7 and 8 Henrietta Street, Covent Garden, W.C.2.

TELEPHONE Temple Bar 3386-7-8

REFERENCE BOOKS

BAILLIÈRE'S NURSES' DICTIONARY

Revised by BARBARA F. CAPE, S.R.N., S.C.M., D.N.

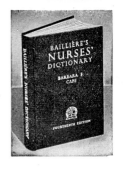

A new edition of this ever-popular dictionary, thoroughly revised and brought up to date. The 25 appendixes of " Essential Information " are a special feature.

Fourteenth Edition. 538 pages, 507 drawings.

6s. 6d. *Postage and packing 9d.*

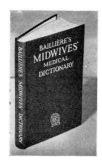

BAILLIÈRE'S MIDWIVES' DICTIONARY

VERA DA CRUZ, S.R.N., S.C.M., S.T.D.

The ideal pocket-sized dictionary for the obstetric nurse " A little mine of invaluable information . . . it really does contain the exact definition wanted in a hurry "— *The Midwives' Chronicle.*

Third Edition. 350 pages, 150 illustrations.

33 appendixes of essential information.

6s. 6d. *Postage and packing 9d.*

BAILLIÈRE'S POCKET BOOK OF WARD INFORMATION

Revised by MARJORIE HOUGHTON, M.B.E., S.R.N., S.C.M., D.N.

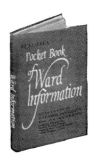

Contents include:
Weights and Measures, Dosage and Solution Strengths, Thermometers Pharmaceutical Preparations, Classification of Drugs, Prescription Abbreviations, Dangerous Drugs, Dosages, Antibiotics, Hormones, Treatment of Poisoning, Sterilization, Disinfectants and Antiseptics, Enemas, X-rays, Maintaining Respiration, Oxygen Therapy, Fluid Balance, Blood Transfusion, Urine Testing, Laboratory Tests, Calories.

Ninth Edition. 224 pages.

6s. 6d. *Postage and packing 9d.*

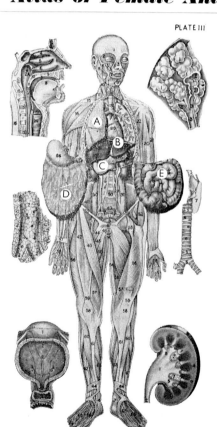

the Male and Female Anatomy are so valuable for they
ail of every part and structure of the human body. Each
ext explaining and teaching the anatomy and physiology
in. × 8½ in. each. By Miss Katharine Armstrong, S.R.N.,

es published"

Atlas of Male Anatomy

*Four coloured and three
black and white plates.*

To study human
anatomy it is essential to
consider both the male
and the female body.
That is why it is
necessary to have two
Atlases. The Male Atlas
is just as important and
essential as the Female
Atlas. See how clearly
in spite of its reduced
size) every detail stands
out in the illustration of
Plate IV on the right,
which is printed in full
colour in the atlas and
shews the vascular
system, the veins and
arteries, the heart in various aspects, the pelvic
contents etc. Plate IV is
another example of "To
see is to learn", and
studied with the simple,
clear explanatory text,
learning becomes easy.
To all who have to
study anatomy Baillière's
Atlases of the Male and
Female body are indis-
pensable.

Postage 1/6.

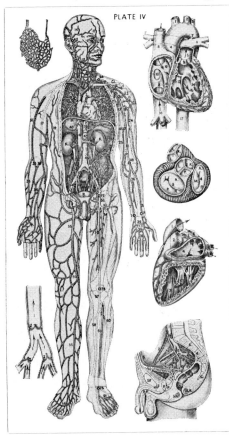

PLATE IV

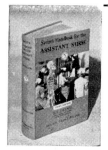

SWIRE'S HANDBOOK FOR THE ASSISTANT NURSE

Revised by R. THORA FARNOL, S.R.N., S.C.M., D.N.

The only textbook of its kind written expressly for the assistant nurse with a full appreciation of her needs derived from practical experience. Covers the syllabus of the G.N.C. and provides a basis of practical knowledge for both training and after-years.

Fourth Edition. In Preparation

A HANDBOOK FOR NURSERY NURSES

ANNE B. MEERING, S.R.N., S.C.M., H.V. CERT.

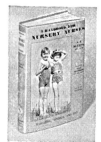

" As a work of reference its value is at once apparent, for it deals with every aspect of child welfare. . . . In fact, the book is . . . all inclusive."—*Nursery Journal*.
" Outstanding . . . thoroughly comprehensive, clearly written and easy for reference."—*Nursery World*.

Third Edition. 576 pages, 111 illus.

22s. 6d. *Postage and packing 1s. 9d.*

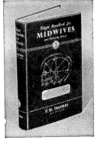

MAYES' HANDBOOK FOR MID-WIVES AND MATERNITY NURSES

Revised by F. D. THOMAS, S.R.N., S.C.M., M.T.D.

" Packed with sound advice and instruction . . . the author's succinct manner of teaching is admirably demonstrated throughout . . . profusely illustrated. Practising midwives will find this handbook a mine of information."—*Nursing Times*.

Sixth Edition. 470 pages, 19 plates and 167 illus.

22s. 6d. *Postage and packing 1s. 9d.*

BERKELEY'S PICTORIAL MIDWIFERY

Revised by D. M. STERN, M.A., M.B., Ch.B., F.R.C.S., F.R.C.O.G.

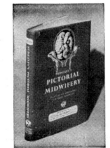

A pictorial survey with excellent illustrations accompanied by clear descriptive text, which will prove invaluable to the pupil midwife, and to the qualified midwife. Really a *must* for any midwife.

Fifth Edition. 176 pages, with 2 coloured plates and 224 drawings

15s. *Postage and packing 1s. 3d.*